Real Medicine In Jesus' Day

COPYRIGHT © Ron McRay, October 2017
Printed in the United States of America

I0769845

Ron McRay
720 W O'Neil Dr Apt 182
Casa Grande AZ 85122
nonelbc@gmail.com
www.eschatologyreview.com

Disclaimer: I am not a medical doctor and you should visit and talk with a health-care provider before you use any information in this book.

Cover photo: copyright Chamille White / 123RF Stock Photo

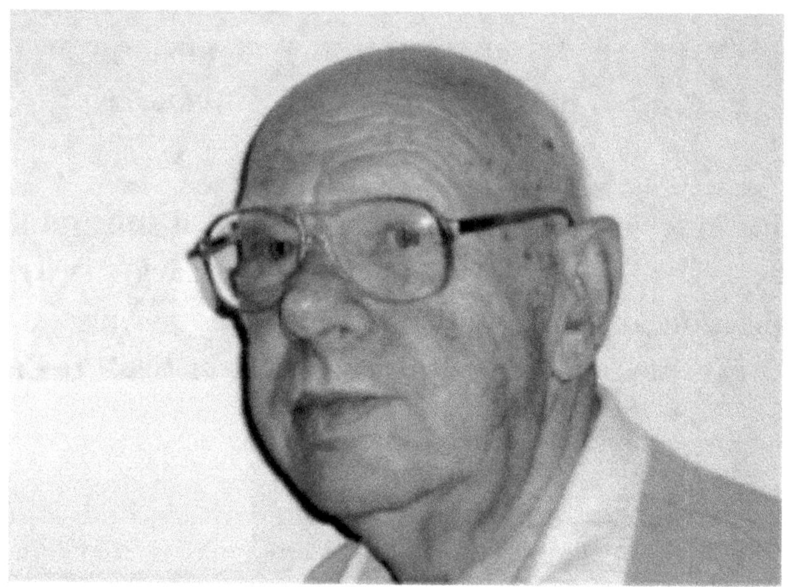

Ron McRay

Thank you for purchasing
"Real Medicine In Jesus' Day"

I would like to give you a special gift

My gift to you is a free audio version of my book
"Are There Three Heavens... Or More?"

<u>Please use the link on the last page to Download Your Bonus Book</u>

This book is just one of my books in the series:

Things That Your Preacher Forgot To Tell You!

Use it to enhance your Bible study

Listen on your way to work or while walking or working in the yard

I hope you enjoy this valuable addition

TABLE OF CONTENTS

CHAPTER ONE 8

    FRANKINCENSE 8

CHAPTER TWO 15

    SECOND OCCURANCE 15

CHAPTER THREE 20

    IN THE "OLD TESTAMENT" 20

CHAPTER FOUR 26

    LEVITICUS 2:1-2 26

CHAPTER FIVE 31

    LEVITICUS 24:7 31

CHAPTER SIX 36

    NUMBERS 5:15 36

CHAPTER SEVEN 49

    1 CHRONICLES 9:29 49

CHAPTER EIGHT 52

    NEHEMIAH 13:5&9 52

CHAPTER NINE 60

    SONG OF SOLOMON 3:6 60

CHAPTER TEN 69

    SONG OF SOLOMON 4:6 69

CHAPTER ELEVEN 73

    SONG OF SOLOMON 4:14 73

CHAPTER TWELVE 79

    ISAIAH 60:6 79

CHAPTER THIRTEEN 86

    JEREMIAH 6:20 86

CHAPTER FOURTEEN 94

    MYRRH 94

CHAPTER FIFTEEN 100

    MARK 15:23 100

CHAPTER SIXTEEN 104

    JOHN 19:39 104

CHAPTER SEVENTEEN 108

    GENESIS 37:25 108

CHAPTER EIGHTEEN 114

    GENESIS 43:11 114

CHAPTER NINETEEN 118

    EXODUS 30:23 118

CHAPTER TWENTY 122

    ESTHER 2:12 122

CHAPTER TWENTY-ONE 133

    SONG OF SOLOMON 1:13 133

CHAPTER TWENTY-TWO 138

    SONG OF SOLOMON 3:6 138

CHAPTER TWENTY-THREE 142

    SONG OF SOLOMON 4:6 & 14 142

CHAPTER TWENTY-FOUR 144

    SONG OF SOLOMON 5:1 & 5 144

CHAPTER TWENTY-FIVE 146

SONG OF SOLOMON 5:13 146

CHAPTER TWENTY SIX 147

GOLD 147

CHAPTER TWENTY Seven 152

GOLDEN 152

CONCLUSION 159

BOOKS BY RON MCRAY 160

FRANKINCENSE

CHAPTER ONE

<u>FRANKINCENSE</u>

The first word that we shall look at is <u>**FRANKINCENSE**</u>. Did you know that the word is used only three times in the *"new testament"*? Did you know that the word is only used in Matthew and Luke? Did you know that it is only used in reference to the magi that came from the east in the childhood of Jesus?

Well, if that is about what you thought, you might be wrong. In the two translations that we shall look, let us first begin with the one in Matthew in the <u>New American Standard Version</u>. The reading is long and in order to get the wise men and Jesus into the passage ...

> *"Then Herod secretly called the magi and determined from them the **exact** time the star appeared. 8 And he sent them to Bethlehem and said, "Go and search carefully for the child; and when you have found him, report to me, so that I too may come and worship him." 9 After hearing the king, they went their way; and the star, which they had seen in the east, went on before them until it came and stood over the place where the child was. 10 When they saw the star, they rejoiced exceedingly with great joy. 11 After coming into the **house**, they saw the child with Mary his mother; and they fell to the ground and worshiped him. Then, opening their treasures, they presented to him gifts of gold, **FRANKINCENSE**, and myrrh. 12 And having been*

warned by Yahweh in a dream not to return to Herod, the magi left for their own country by another way" [Matthew 2:7-12].

There are differences between that passage and the one in the King James Version which follows – compare it. The underscore words are different ...

*"Then Herod, when he had privily called the wise men, inquired of them diligently what time the star appeared. 8 And he sent them to Bethlehem, and said, Go and search diligently for the young child; and when ye have found him, bring me word again, that I may come and worship him also. 9 When they had heard the king, they departed; and, lo, the star, which they saw in the east, went before them, till it came and stood over where the young child was. 10 When they saw the star, they rejoiced with exceeding great joy. 11 And when they were come into the house, they saw the young child with Mary his mother, and fell down, and worshipped him: and when they had opened their treasures, they presented unto him gifts; gold, and **FRANKINCENSE**, and myrrh. 12 And being warned of Yahweh in a dream that they should not return to Herod, they departed into their own country another way*" [Matthew 2:7-12].

Boy - that was a lot of work for me to handle the two verses and show how they differed! Both have **FRANKINCENSE** and that was the main thrust of the verse and this book. Of the many translations that I have, they are all different. When you compare the two verses, the **magi were the wise men** and there is an obvious difference between a **baby and a young child** in those two verses. Actually, the Greek verses coincide with the

King James Version in this case. This revelation that the magi had, could have come through some contact with Israelite scholars who had migrated to the East with copies of the *"old testament"* manuscripts. Many feel the magi's comments reflected knowledge of Balaam's prophecy concerning the *"star"* that would *"come out of Jacob"* (Numbers 24:17). Whatever the source, they came to Jerusalem to worship the newborn king of the Israelites. We do not know how many magi there were. From the three gifts listed in Matthew 2:11, some people have **assumed** there were three kings from the Orient, though this is not certain. But when their **caravan** arrived in Jerusalem, there were **enough of them to trouble the whole city**. The magi must have come with quite an entourage for the whole city to notice them. *"Magi"* (*not* *"wise* *men"*) were astrologers whose divinatory skills were widely respected in the Greco-Roman world; astrology had become popular through the *"science"* of the East, and everyone agreed that the best astrologers lived in the East. Be very careful in your studies for our **traditions** as handed down. All of these are, at the best, **precarious suppositions**.

The people of the east never approached the presence of kings and great personages, without a present in their hands. This custom is often noticed in the *"old testament,"* and still prevails in the East and in some of the newly discovered South Sea Islands.

Some have those gifts to be emblematic of the Divinity, regal office and the manhood of Jesus …

> *"They offered him **INCENSE** as Yahweh; gold as their king; and myrrh, as united to a human body, subject to suffering and death."*

No doubt but that they offered to Jesus the things which were in most esteem among themselves; and which were productions of their own country. The gold was probably a very providential supply, as on it, **possibly** likely, they subsisted while in Egypt. But in this paragraph, instead of the two translations using **FRANKINCENSE**, this paragraph uses the word **INCENSE**. Most people know how to pronounce **FRANKINCENSE** but really do not know what it means. In short it means …

> *"**FRANKINCENSE**, also called olibanum, is an aromatic resin used in **INCENSE** and **perfumes**, obtained from trees of the genus Boswellia in the family Burseraceae, particularly Boswellia sacra (syn: B. carteri, B. bhaw-dajiana), B. frereana, B. serrata (B. thurifera, Indian frankincense), and B. papyrifera."*

Jesus was an Israelite and they always had incense. So, in this paragraph, the word **FRANKINCENSE** is used as **INCENSE**. The English word is derived from the old French *"franc encens"* (i.e., **high quality INCENSE**). There are four main species of Boswellia that produce true **FRANKINCENSE**. Resin from each of the four is available in various grades. The grades depend on the time of harvesting; the resin is hand-sorted for quality. I understand that most of the **FRANKINCENSE** today comes from a country called Somalia. You can order capsules of Boswellia at the health food store.

FRANKINCENSE is tapped from the rough but hardy trees by slashing the bark and permitting the resin to bleed out and harden. These hardened resins are called *"tears"*. There are several species and varieties of **FRANKINCENSE** trees, each producing a slightly different type of resin. Differences in soil and climate create even more diversity of the resin, even within the same species. Boswellia sacra trees are considered unusual for their ability to grow in environments so unforgiving that they sometimes grow out of solid rock, which process is unknown. This growth prevents it from being ripped from the rock during violent storms. The trees start producing resin when they are about eight to ten years old. Tapping is done two to three times a year with the final taps producing the best *"tears"* due to their higher aromatic terpene, sesquiterpene and diterpene content. Generally speaking, the more opaque resins are the best quality. Fine resin is produced in Somalia, from which the Roman Catholic Church purchases most of its stock.

FRANKINCENSE tree populations were declining in 2016 A.D. due to over-exploitation. Heavily tapped trees produce seeds that germinate at only 16% while seeds of trees that had not been tapped germinate at more than 80%. Also, burning, grazing and attacks by the longhorn beetle have reduced the tree population. Conversion (*clearing*) of **FRANKINCENSE** woodlands to agriculture is also a major threat.

I think that it is time to go back to Matthew 2:11 again. Go back up and reread this verse and then begin to make some comparisons. Some problems begin to occur. First, when the wise men entered and saw Jesus, he was **not in a manger** but a house. He was **no longer a baby**, he was a young child. In all probability, Jesus, along with his parents, had made that same trip each year due to a lawful command that both Joseph and Mary had to **enroll in a census**. It was probably about two years since Jesus was born when Matthew 2 pertained. There is another chapter in the Bible that tells of Jesus' birth. It is Luke chapter one which is different than Matthew. If you will read that, you will begin to ask yourself some more questions that you have not heard before. But I do not have the time and space to deal with those 2 chapters in this book.

It was probably not the place where Jesus was born; it was probably the place where they lived at that time. *"Falling down"* was the usual way of showing respect or homage among the Israelites [Esther 8:3; Job 1:20; Daniel 3:7; Psalms 72:11; Isaiah 46:6]. The wise men did homage to Jesus (*worshipped him*) as king of the Israelites. He was the king of the **Israelites**. The magi opened their treasures which they had brought, or the boxes, etc., in which they had brought their gold, etc.. The gifts were presented to him as king of the Israelites, because they supposed he was to be a distinguished prince and conqueror. It was customary in the East to show respect for persons of distinction by making presents or offerings of this kind (Genesis 32:14; 43:11; 1 Samuel 10:27; 1 Kings 10:2; Psalms 72:10-15). This custom is still common in the East, and it is unusual to approach a person of distinguished rank without a valuable present.

FRANKINCENSE is found in the East Indies, but chiefly in Arabia; and hence it has been supposed probable that the wise men came from Arabia. **Myrrh** was also a production of Arabia, and was obtained from a tree in the same manner as **FRANKINCENSE**. **Myrrh** was an ingredient of the holy ointment (Exodus 30:23).

CHAPTER TWO

SECOND OCCURENCE

The next passage that comes in the *"new testament"* is Revelation 18. It also is a little longer in order for the passage to make sense. The first passage is from the <u>King James Version</u> …

<u>"Therefore shall her plagues come in one day, death, and mourning, and famine; and she shall be utterly burned with fire: for strong is the Lord Yahweh who judgeth her. 9 And the kings of the earth, who have committed fornication and lived deliciously with her, shall bewail her, and lament for her, when they shall see the smoke of her burning, 10 Standing afar off for the fear of her torment, saying, Alas, alas, that great city Babylon, that mighty city! for in one hour is thy judgment come. 11 And the merchants of the earth shall weep and mourn over her; for no man buyeth their merchandise any more: 12 The merchandise of gold, and silver, and precious stones, and of pearls, and fine linen, and purple, and silk, and scarlet, and all thyine wood, and all manner vessels of ivory, and all manner vessels of most precious wood, and of brass, and iron, and marble, 13 And cinnamon, and odours, and ointments, and</u> **<u>FRANKINCENSE</u>**<u>*, and wine, and oil, and fine flour, and wheat, and beasts, and sheep, and horses, and chariots, and slaves, and souls of men. 14 And the fruits that thy soul lusted after are departed from thee, and all things which were dainty and goodly are departed from thee, and thou*</u>

*shalt find them no more at all. 15 The merchants of these things, which were made rich by her, shall stand afar off for the fear of her torment, weeping and wailing, 16 And saying, alas, alas, that great city, that was clothed in fine linen, and purple, and scarlet, and decked with gold, and precious stones, and pearls! 17 For in one hour so great riches is come to nought. And every shipmaster, and all the company in ships, and sailors, and as many as trade by sea, stood afar off, 18 And cried when they saw the smoke of her burning, saying, What city is like unto this great city! 19 And they cast dust on their heads, and cried, weeping and wailing, saying, Alas, alas, that great city, wherein were made rich all that had ships in the sea by reason of her costliness! for in one hour is she made desolate. 20 Rejoice over her, thou heaven, and ye holy **apostles** and prophets; for Yahweh hath avenged you on her. 21 And a mighty angel took up a stone like a great millstone, and cast it into the sea, saying, Thus with violence shall that great city Babylon be thrown down, and shall be found no more at all"* [Revelation 18:8-21].

Among those individuals who believe in Yahweh, there are more people who take Revelation to have been written after 96 A.D.. But, if you have such feelings **as I once did**, you are as wrong as I was for 35 years of preaching and another 10 years of studying the Bible for me to at least understand the basics of the book of Revelation. Please join me – you will feel much, much better and you will learn more. Think seriously now.

Probably, Revelation was written before any other *"new testament"* book was written. There are many references in the *"new testament"* that **proves** that the book of Revelation was written **before** 74 A.D. but no exact date. Accept what I just said whether you agree or not and continue studying till you can see at least that much. If you can do that much; you will see the type and antitypes in the book. In our paragraph at hand, the type of Babylon is used for **PHYSICAL JERUSALEM** being destroyed in 70 A.D.. If I had time and space I could probably write about five books on this one chapter. However, that is not the subject of this book. So, let us stay with the subject which is **FRANKINCENSE**.

Regarding production, **FRANKINCENSE** is often prepared inside a censer, such as the *meerschaum dabqaad* traditionally used in Somalia and Djibouti. Estimates of the current annual world production of **FRANKINCENSE** vary, but generally are around several thousand tons. More than 82% of the product comes from Somalia, with some **FRANKINCENSE** also gathered in adjacent Southern Arabia and Ethiopia, and other central African countries.

FRANKINCENSE has been traded on the Arabian Peninsula and in North Africa for more than 5,000 years. A mural depicting sacks of **FRANKINCENSE** traded from the Land of Punt adorns the walls of the temple of ancient Egyptian Queen Hatshepsut, who died circa 1,458 B.C..

FRANKINCENSE was one of the consecrated incenses (*HaKetoret*) described in the Hebrew Bible and Talmud. The

FRANKINCENSE of the Israelites, as well as of the Greeks and Romans, is also called Olibanum (*from the Hebrew חלבנה*). *"Old testament"* references report it in trade from Sheba. It was offered on a specialized **incense** altar in the time when the Tabernacle was located in the First and Second Jerusalem Temples. It was an important component of the Temple service in Jerusalem. It is mentioned in the Hebrew Bible book of Exodus 30:34, where it is named *"lebonah"* in the Biblical Hebrew, meaning "*white*" in Hebrew. It was one of the ingredients in the perfume of the sanctuary and was used as an accompaniment of the meal-offering. When burnt, it emitted a fragrant odor, and the **incense** was a symbol of the Divine name and an emblem of prayer. It was often associated with **myrrh** and with it was made an offering to the infant Jesus. A special "*pure*" kind was presented with the showbread.

FRANKINCENSE was reintroduced to Europe by Frankish Crusaders. There is a reference to the milky sap tapped from the Boswellia tree. Some have also postulated that the name comes from the Arabic term for "*Oil of Lebanon,*" since Lebanon was the place where the resin was sold and traded with Europeans. The lost city of Ubar, sometimes identified with Irem in what is now the town of Shisr in Oman, is believed to have been a center of the **FRANKINCENSE** trade along the recently rediscovered "***Incense** Road.*" Ubar was rediscovered in the early 1990's and is now under archaeological excavation.

The Greek historian Herodotus was familiar with **FRANKINCENSE** and knew it was harvested from trees in southern Arabia. He reported that the gum was dangerous to harvest because of venomous snakes that lived in the trees. He goes on to describe the method used by the Arabs to get around this problem; that being, the burning of the gum of the tree whose smoke would drive the snakes away.

The word is only used two times in the *"new testament"* which I have listed above. Next, we will go to the use of the word in the *"old testament."*

CHAPTER THREE

IN THE "OLD TESTAMENT"

FRANKINCENSE was first used or at least spoken about very early in Israelite history and connected with the tent of meeting where Yahweh met with the Israelite people. Here is the passage in the <u>New American Standard Version</u> …

> *"Then the Lord said to Moses, "Take for yourself spices, stacte and onycha and galbanum, spices with pure **FRANKINCENSE**; there shall be an equal part of each. 35 "With it you shall make **incense, a perfume**, the work of a perfumer, salted, pure, and holy. 36 "You shall beat some of it very fine, and put part of it **before the testimony in the tent of meeting** where I will meet with you; it shall be most holy to you. 37 "The **incense** which you shall make, you shall not make in the same proportions for yourselves; it shall be holy to you for the Lord. 38 "Whoever shall make any like it, to use as perfume, shall be cut off from his people" [Exodus 30:34-38].*

We have just looked at the <u>NASV</u>, so before we get any further, let us look at the same verses in the <u>King James Version</u> …

> "And the Lord said unto Moses, Take unto thee **sweet** spices, stacte, and onycha, and galbanum; **these sweet spices** with pure **FRANKINCENSE; of each shall there be a like weight. 35 And thou shalt make it** a perfume, **a confection after the art of the**

apothecary, tempered together, pure and holy. 36 And thou shalt beat some of it very **small, and put of it** before the testimony in the tabernacle of the **congregation**, where I will meet with thee - it shall be unto you most holy. 37 And as for the **perfume** which thou shalt make, ye shall not make to yourselves **according to the composition thereof**: it shall be unto thee holy for the Lord. 38 Whosoever shall make like unto that, **to smell thereto**, shall even be cut off from his people" [Exodus 30:34-38].

As you look at all of the high-lighted words in the KJV, the passage teaches about the same. However, there is much misunderstanding in the words **perfume** and **incense**. One uses the word **sweet** while the other one does not use any word. One uses **equal part** while the other one uses **weight**. Search through the two verses as to the difference of the other parts. The word **weight** has been added to the *"old testament"* in these verses. Other than that, the King James Version seems to be the better of the two translations.

If you are not very familiar with the Bible, especially the *"old testament,"* you will find many words of which you are not familiar – like *"stacte and onycha."* But, I will not spend any time on those words and try to stay with the subject of **FRANKINCENSE**. However, I will talk about the three words in this passage. The holy perfume was compounded from the following ingredients: Stacte is supposed to be the same with what was afterward called *"the balm of Jericho."* Stacte is the gum which spontaneously flows from the tree which produces

myrrh. Onycha is the external crust of the shell-fish purpura or murex, and is the basis of the principal **perfumes** made in the East Indies. Galbanum rises with a ligneous stalk from eight to ten feet and is garnished with leaves at each joint. The top of the stock is terminated by yellow flowers, which are succeeded by oblong channeled seeds, which have a thin membrane or wing on their border. When any part of the plant is broken, there issues out a little thin milk of a cream color. The gummy resinous juice which proceeds from this plant is what is commonly called galbanum, from the *"chelbenah"* of the Hebrews. Added to those three things, the Lord wanted **PURE FRANKINCENSE**. This was the most important of the aromatic gums. Like **myrrh**, it was regarded by itself as a precious perfume and it was used unmixed with other substances in some of the rites of the Law of Moses. The tree from which it is obtained is not found in Arabia, and it was most likely imported from India. The tree is now known as the Boswellia serrata and grows abundantly in the highlands of India. The **FRANKINCENSE** of commerce is a different substance, the resin of the spruce and of some other kinds of fir. Salt was to be added to the mixture to give forth a **white smoke**, and to add to the **fragrance**. **FRANKINCENSE** is from a root meaning "*whiteness*," referring to the milky color of the fresh juice – which is found in about 20 verses in the Bible. The word is translated in the last six references as **INCENSE** in the <u>King James Version</u>, but **correctly** in the Revised Version

(*British and American*). Some of the trees grow to a considerable height and send down their roots to extraordinary depths. The gum is obtained by incising the bark, and is collected in yellowish, semitransparent tears, readily pulverized; it has a nauseous taste. It is used for making **incense** for burning in churches and in Indian temples, as it was among the Israelites. **FRANKINCENSE** comes in many types, and its quality is based on color, purity, aroma, age and shape. Silver and Hojari are generally considered the highest grades of **FRANKINCENSE**. **FRANKINCENSE** is used in perfumery and aromatherapy. It is also an ingredient that is sometimes used in skincare. The essential oil is obtained by steam distillation of the dry resin. Some of the smells of the **FRANKINCENSE** smoke are products of pyrolysis. **FRANKINCENSE** is used in many churches, including the Eastern Orthodox, Oriental Orthodox and Catholic churches. Christian and Islamic Abrahamic faiths have all used **FRANKINCENSE** mixed with oils to anoint newborn infants, initiates and members entering into new phases of their spiritual lives.

Conversely, the spread of *"Christianity"* depressed the market for **FRANKINCENSE** during the 4th century A.D.. Desertification made the caravan routes across the *"Empty Quarter"* of the Arabian Peninsula more difficult. Additionally, increased raiding by the nomadic Parthians in the Near East caused the **FRANKINCENSE** trade to dry up after 300 A.D..

Salt, in fact, was to be added to all the offerings (Leviticus 2:13). The **incense** was to be placed in front of the Testimony (*i.e., the ark*), which probably means that it was to be **burned on the altar of incense** which was in front of the curtain to the most holy place. This **incense**, like the anointing oil, was **exclusively for tabernacle use**. If it was accepted, it was called a sweet savor; if the contrary, it was called *"a stink in the nostrils,"* or *"a stinking savor."*

The altar of **incense** was made of acacia wood and **overlaid with gold**, and was a foot and a half square and three feet high. It was the tallest piece of furniture in the holy place. It had an ornamental gold rim ("*crown*") around the top and golden "*horns*" at each corner. It stood before the veil that separated the holy of holies from the holy place, and the priest burned **incense** on it each morning and evening when he trimmed the lamps. In order to please Yahweh and not be in danger of death, the priest had to use not only the right fire on the altar but also the prescribed mixture of spices for the **incense**. Nadab and Abihu tried to worship Yahweh with "*false fire*" and were killed. Any Israelite who tried to duplicate this special **incense** for his own personal use would he cut off, which meant death. Once a year, on the Day of Atonement, the priest had to apply blood to the **incense** altar in order to make it ceremonially clean before Yahweh (Exodus 30:10 - Exodus 30:22-38).

This was prepared once a year (*the Israelites say*), a pound for each day of the year, and three pounds over for the **day of atonement**. When it was used, it was to be **beaten very small**; thus it pleased the Lord to **bruise the Redeemer** when he offered himself for a sacrifice of a sweet-smelling savor.

CHAPTER FOUR

<u>LEVITICUS 2:1-2</u>

*"Now when anyone presents a grain offering as an offering to the Lord, his offering shall be of fine flour, and he shall pour oil on it and put **FRANKINCENSE** on it. 2 He shall then bring it to Aaron's sons the priests; and shall take from it his handful of its fine flour and of its oil with all of its **FRANKINCENSE**. And the priest shall offer it up in smoke as its memorial portion on the altar, an offering by fire of a soothing aroma to the Lord. 3 The remainder of the grain offering belongs to Aaron and his sons: a thing most holy, of the offerings to the Lord by fire"* [Leviticus 2:1-3 – NASU].

The word **FRANKINCENSE** is used twice in this series of verses. Let us look also at the <u>King James Version</u> ...

*"And when any will offer a **meat** offering unto the Lord, his offering shall be of fine flour; and he shall pour oil upon it, and put **FRANKINCENSE** thereon: 2 And he shall bring it to Aaron's sons the priests: and he shall take thereout his handful of the flour thereof, and of the oil thereof, with all the **FRANKINCENSE** thereof; and the priest shall **burn the memorial** of it upon the altar, to be an offering made by fire, of a **sweet** savour unto the Lord: 3 And the **remnant of the meat offering** shall be Aaron's and his sons'; it is a thing most holy of the offerings of the Lord made by fire"* [Leviticus 2:1-3].

I underlined about four lines that you can go to the two verses and compare them. **Was it (*they*) a meal offering or a meat**

offering? Everything in the verses seem to indicate a **_meal_** offering rather than a *"meat"* offering. Would you believe that **flour** indicated a *"baked"* cake rather than there was an animal slaughtered?

Men have remarked that there are five kinds of the flour mentioned in this chapter …

    1. Simple flour or meal, Leviticus 2:1.

    2. Cakes and wafers, or whatever was baked in the oven, Leviticus 2:4.

    3. Cakes baked in the pan, Leviticus 2:6.

    4. Cakes baked on the frying-pan, or probably, a grid-iron, Leviticus 2:7.

    5. Green ears of corn (*grain*) parched, Leviticus 2:14.

All these were offered **without** honey or leaven, but accompanied with wine, oil and **FRANKINCENSE**. The green ears of corn dried by the fire, etc., was properly the gratitude-offering for a good seed time, and the prospect of a plentiful harvest. This appears to have been the offering brought by Cain.

The flour, whether of wheat, rice, barley, rye or any other grain used for an **ailment**, was in all likelihood equally proper; for we elsewhere in the Bible find the flour of barley or barley meal, is called acceptable. It is plain to me that in this passage, no animal was here included, though in other places it is possible to include both kinds; but in general, it was not a bloody offering, nor used by way of atonement or expiation, but merely in a eucharistic way, expressing gratitude to Yahweh for the produce of the soil.

It is such an offering as what we might call *"natural religion"* and might be reasonably expected to suggest - but alas!! so far lost is mankind, that even thankfulness to Yahweh for the fruits of the earth must be taught by a divine revelation for in the heart of men even the seeds of gratitude are not found, till sown there by the hand of divine grace.

Offerings of different kinds of grain, flour, bread, fruits, etc., are the most ancient among the pagan nations, and even the people of Yahweh have had them from the beginning. There is the idea that those gratitude-offerings originated with agriculture ...

> *"In the most ancient times men lived by hunting, etc., for the sword was considered to be more honorable than the plow; but when they sowed their fields, they dedicated the first-fruits of their harvest to Yahweh, to whom the ancients attributed the art of agriculture, and to whom burnt-offerings of corn (grain) were made, according to immemorial usages."*

Yahweh required nothing here which was not in common use **for nourishment**; but He commanded that those things should be offered with such articles as might give them the most exquisite relish, such as salt, oil and wine and that the flour should be of the finest and purest kind. The ancient Israelites seem to have made much use of meal formed into a paste with milk, and sometimes with water. The priests kept in the temples a certain mixture of flour mingled with oil and wine, which they called _health_, and which they used as a kind of charm **against sickness**. After they had finished their sacrifices, they generally threw some flour upon the fire, mingled with oil and wine, which was the ordinary sacrifice of the poor.

It was remarked that there was neither oil nor **incense** offered with the sin and **jealousy** offerings, because they were **not offerings of memorial**, but such as brought iniquities to Yahweh's remembrance, which were neither gracious nor sweet-smelling before the Lord. In this case, a handful only was burnt, the rest was reserved for the priest's use, but all the **FRANKINCENSE** was burned, because from it the priest could derive no advantage.

FRANKINCENSE has been used in traditional **medicine** for generations, even farther back than the beginning of the Law of Moses. **FRANKINCENSE resin is edible** and is used in traditional medicines in Africa and Asia for digestion and healthy skin. For internal consumption, it is recommended that **FRANKINCENSE** be translucent, with no black or brown impurities. It is often light yellow with a very slight greenish tint. It is often chewed like gum, but it is stickier. It also has been used for hundreds of years for **treating arthritis, healing wounds, strengthening the female hormone system and purifying the air**. In Somali, Ethiopian, Arabian and Indian cultures, it is suggested that burning **FRANKINCENSE daily** in the house **brings good health**. **FRANKINCENSE oil** can also be used for relief from **stings such as scorpion stings**.

CHAPTER FIVE

<u>LEVITICUS 24:7</u>

This is Leviticus 24:5-9 in the <u>New American Standard Version</u> ...

> *"Then you shall take fine flour and **bake** twelve cakes with it; two-tenths of an ephah shall be in each cake. 6 "You shall set them in two rows, six to a row, on the pure **gold** table before the Lord. 7 "You shall put pure **FRANKINCENSE** on each row that it may be a **memorial** portion for the bread, even an offering by fire to the Lord. 8 "**Every sabbath day** he shall set it in order before the Lord continually; it is **an everlasting covenant** for the **SONS OF ISRAEL**. 9 "It shall be for Aaron and his sons, and they shall eat it in a holy place; for it is most holy to him from the Lord's offerings by fire, his portion forever."*

As is usual, let us look at the same series of verses from the <u>King James Version</u>, that is, Leviticus 24:5-9 ...

> *"And thou shalt take fine flour, and bake twelve cakes thereof: two tenth **deals** shall be in one cake. 6 And thou shalt set them in two rows, six on a row, upon the pure table before the Lord. 7 And thou shalt put pure **FRANKINCENSE** upon each row, that it may be **on the bread for a memorial**, even an offering made by fire unto the Lord. 8 Every sabbath he shall set it in order before the Lord continually, being taken from the children of Israel by an everlasting covenant. 9*

> *And it shall be Aaron's and his sons'; and they shall eat it in **the** holy place: for it is most holy unto him of the offerings of the Lord made by fire **by a perpetual statute.**"*

As to these first passages, please go to both the <u>NASV</u> and the <u>KJV</u> and look for any differences. As far as the originals are concerned, they both are about equal, both having words that are not in the original. Let us look at the verses.

Verse 5 no doubt is the table of shew-bread in the tabernacle on which was **<u>unleavened</u>** bread. It was also called "*the bread of the Presence.*" Each cake represented the offering of a tribe. They were probably placed in **two piles** (<u>NIV</u>, 2 rows). **Incense** was placed on the table beside the bread to be burned on the altar as a memorial portion each Sabbath when the old bread was replaced and **given to the priests as their regular share**. On each (*row*) pile of cakes some **<u>FRANKINCENSE</u>** was strewed, which, being burnt, led to the showbread being called "*an offering made by fire.*" The preparation of the shew-bread and the use to be made of it are **described here for the first time**; though it had already been offered by the congregation at the consecration of the tabernacle, and placed by Moses upon the table.

Some infer that this showbread, which was set on the table on the Sabbath, was intended as **<u>a memorial</u>** of the manna wherewith they were fed in the wilderness.

Each cake weighed a little over six pounds. The Levites were in charge with making the loaves. Each cake represented the offering of one tribe of the children of Israel. Each cake represented the offering of a tribe. Note this passage which you have probably overlooked ...

> _"You shall take **two onyx stones** and engrave on them the names of the sons of Israel, 10 **six of their names on the one stone and the names of the remaining six on the other stone, according to their birth**. 11 "As a jeweler engraves a signet, you shall engrave the two stones according to the names of the sons of Israel; you shall set them in filigree settings of gold. 12 "You shall put the two stones on the shoulder pieces of the ephod, as stones of memorial for the sons of Israel, and **Aaron shall bear their names** before the Lord on his two shoulders for a memorial" [Exodus 28:9-13]._

But let us not forget the main part of this book – **FRANKINCENSE**. An enriched extract of _"Indian **FRANKINCENSE**"_ (usually Boswellia serrata) was used in a randomized, double-blinded, placebo-controlled study of patients with osteoarthritis. **Patients receiving the extract showed significant improvement in their arthritis in as little as seven days. The compound caused no major adverse effects and, according to the study authors, is safe for human consumption and long-term use**. In a study published in 2009, it was reported that _"**FRANKINCENSE** oil appears to distinguish **cancerous from normal bladder cells and suppress cancer cell viability**."_ A 2012 study in _"healthy"_ volunteers determined that exposure to 11-keto-β-boswellic acid

(KBA), a lead boswellic acid in the novel solubilized **FRANKINCENSE** extract Boswelan, is increased when taken with food. However, simulations based on a two-compartment pharmacokinetic model with single first-order absorption phase proposed that the observed food interaction loses its relevance for the simulated repeated-dose scenario. In a 2012 study, researchers found that the "*behavioral effect [of insensole actetate] was concomitant to reduced serum corticosterone levels, dose-dependent down-regulation of corticotropin releasing factor and up-regulation of brain derived neurotrophic factor transcripts IV and VI expression in the hippocampus. These data suggest that IA modulates the hypothalamic–pituitary–adrenal (HPA) axis and influences hippocampal gene expression, leading to beneficial behavioral effects supporting its potential as a novel treatment of depressive-like disorders*."

In 2013, Leicester University researchers announced findings that AKBA (acetyl-11-keto-beta-boswellic acid), a chemical compound in the resin, has **cancer-killing** properties and **has the potential to destroy ovarian cancer cells**. The lead researcher from the University's Department of Cancer Studies and Molecular Medicine announced the findings after a year studying the AKBA compound with ovarian cancer cell lines in vitro that showed it is effective at **killing late stage cancer cells**. Kamla Al-Salmani noted that among surprising findings were that some cells that had become resistant to chemotherapy were killed during the in vitro study. The efficacy of AKBA as a potential **medicine** for treatment of *"cancers (colon, breast and prostate)"* has been tested. The results are based on the preliminary and unverified findings of the laboratory study, which marked the first study to identify an ability to fight ovarian cancer. It is in early stages and, as of 2014, yet to be published in a peer-reviewed journal.

The use of **FRANKINCENSE** and **MYRRH** were apparently given to Jesus for **medicine**. The wise men evidently knew more than scientists do today.

CHAPTER SIX

<u>NUMBERS 5:15</u>

The following series of verses consist of the unfaithfulness of a wife in Israel. I will quote only the verses from the <u>New American Standard Version</u> (*and not quote from the <u>KJV</u>) ...*

> *<u>"Then the Lord spoke to Moses, saying, 12 "Speak to the sons of</u> **<u>Israel</u>** <u>and say to them, 'If any man's wife goes astray and is</u> <u>unfaithful to him, 13 and a</u> **<u>man has intercourse with her</u>** <u>and it is</u> <u>hidden from the eyes of her husband and she is</u> **<u>undetected</u>**<u>,</u> <u>although she has defiled herself, and there is no witness against her</u> <u>and she has not been caught in the act, 14 if a spirit of jealousy</u> <u>comes over him and he is jealous of his wife when she has defiled</u> <u>herself, or if a spirit of jealousy comes over him and he is jealous of</u> <u>his wife when she has not defiled herself, 15 the man shall then</u> <u>bring his wife to the priest, and shall bring as an offering for her one-</u> <u>tenth of an ephah of barley meal; he shall not pour oil on it nor put</u> <u>FRANKINCENSE on it, for it is a grain offering of jealousy, a grain</u> <u>offering of memorial, a reminder of iniquity"</u>* [Numbers 5:11-15].

Whether the wife is guilty or not, this was the rule for the Israelites. Even though **<u>FRANKINCENSE</u>** is mentioned in this oath, I am sure that you would like to see the continuation of this chapter, so here it is ...

> *<u>"16 'Then the</u> **<u>priest shall bring her near and have her stand before</u>** **<u>the Lord,</u>** <u>17 and the priest shall take holy water in an earthenware</u>*

*vessel; and he shall take some of the dust that is on the floor of the tabernacle and put it into the water. 18 'The priest shall then have the woman stand before the Lord and **let the hair of the woman's head go loose**, and place the grain offering of memorial in her hands, which is the grain offering of jealousy, and in the hand of the priest is to be **the water of bitterness that brings a curse**. 19 'The priest shall have her take an **oath** and shall say to the woman, "If no man has lain with you and if you have not gone astray into uncleanness, being under the authority of your husband, be immune to this water of bitterness that brings a curse; 20 if you, however, have gone astray, being under the authority of your husband, and if you have defiled yourself and a man other than your husband has had intercourse with you" 21 (then the priest shall have the woman swear with the oath of the curse, and the priest shall say to the woman), "the Lord make you a curse and an oath among your people by the Lord's making **your thigh waste away and your abdomen swell**; 22 and this water that brings a curse shall go into your stomach, and make your abdomen swell and your thigh waste away." And the woman shall say, "Amen. Amen." 23 'The priest shall then write these curses on a scroll, and he shall wash them off into the water of bitterness. 24 'Then he shall make the woman drink the water of bitterness that brings a curse, so that the water which brings a curse will go into her and cause bitterness. 25 'The priest shall take the grain offering of jealousy from the woman's hand, and he shall wave the grain offering before the Lord and bring it to the altar; 26 and the priest shall take a handful of the grain offering as its memorial offering and offer it up in smoke on the altar, and afterward he shall make the woman drink the water. 27 'When he has made her drink the water, then it shall come about, if she has defiled herself and has been unfaithful to her husband, that the* *water which brings a curse will go into her and cause bitterness, and her abdomen will swell and her thigh will waste away, and the woman will become a curse among her people. 28 'But if the woman has not defiled herself and is clean, she will then be free and conceive children. 29 **This is the law of jealousy**: when a wife, being under the authority of her husband, goes astray and defiles herself, 30 or when a spirit of jealousy comes over a man and he is jealous of his wife, he shall then make the woman stand before the Lord, and the priest shall apply all this law to her. 31 'Moreover, the man will be free from guilt, **but that woman shall bear her guilt**.'"* [Numbers 5:16-31].

I think that the addition of these verses will explain the curse for the undetected harlot, so I will not spend much time on it. There is one part of which I will speak. The women of Israel always kept their hair **up on top of her head**. Only when she is alone with her husband could she put it down. **Are women to practice such today**? It does not refer to a veil. What is meant by these expressions cannot be easily ascertained. *"Yaareek"* signifies literally, <u>thy thigh to fall</u>. Since the thigh, feet etc., were used among the Hebrews delicately to express the parts which nature conceals, the expression here is probably to be understood in this sense, and the falling down of the thigh here must mean something similar to the falling down of the womb, which might be a natural effect of the abdomen. That seems to be more the case when Yahweh says that if she had been faithful, she could have children. There is no place in the Bible where anyone had been put this trial of ordeal. Yahweh's threat was enough!

This is called the trial of jealousy. Since the crime of adultery is especially defiling and destructive of the very foundations of social order, the whole subject is dealt with at a length proportionate to its importance. This mode of trial, like several other ordinances, was adopted by Moses from existing and **probably** very ancient and widely spread institutions. The offering was to be of the **cheapest** and coarsest kind, barley, representing the abused condition of the suspected woman. It was, like the sin-offering, to be made **without** oil and **FRANKINCENSE**, the symbols of grace and acceptableness. The woman herself stood with head uncovered in token of her shame. In the covenant community of Israel - adultery, like ceremonial uncleanness and trespass against one's brother or sister (v-6), was symptomatic of unfaithfulness to the Lord. It therefore could not be tolerated as either a breach of the relationship of husband and wife (Exodus 20:14) or as the expression of covenant infidelity (Ezekiel 16). If a man suspected his wife of adultery, he was to take her before the priest whether he had proof or not. Since adultery also was a sin against Yahweh, the appropriate offering of **barley flour** was to be taken to the priest and offered before the Lord. The purpose of the offering was to draw attention to guilt.

Generally speaking, the person who committed a trespass against another had to confess it and make restitution. It was not enough just to confess the sin and say, "*I'm sorry,*" and then bring a trespass offering to the priest. The offender had to pay the injured party (*or a relative, or the priest*) an amount of money equivalent to the loss incurred and add to it another 20 per-cent. In this way, the Lord taught His people that sin is costly and hurts people, and that true repentance demands honest restitution. But another factor was involved. Israel was about to confront their enemies, and there could be no unity in the army if the people were in conflict with one another because of unresolved offenses. The soldiers would be alienated from each other and from the Lord, and that could lead to defeat. True unity begins with everybody being right with Yahweh and with each other.

If a man's wife went aside and was guilty of unfaithfulness towards him through a (*another*) man having lain with her with "*emissio seminis,*" and it was hidden from the eyes of her husband, on account of her having defiled herself secretly, and there being no witness against her, and her not having been taken (*in the act*); but if, for all that, a spirit of jealousy came upon him, and he was jealous of his wife, and she was defiled, or she was not defiled; the man was to take his wife to the priest, and bring as her sacrificial gift, on her account, the tenth of an ephah of barley meal, without putting oil or incense, "*for it is a meat-offering of jealousy, a meat-offering of memory, to bring iniquity to remembrance.*" As the woman's crime, of which her husband accused her, was naturally denied by herself, and was neither to be supported by witnesses nor proven by her being taken in the very act, the only way left to determine whether there was any foundation or not for the spirit of jealousy excited in her husband, and to prevent an unrighteous severance of the divinely appointed marriage, was to let the thing be decided by the verdict of Yahweh Himself. To this end, the man was to bring his wife to the priest with a sacrificial gift, which is expressly called *"qaar-baanaah,"* her offering, brought "*on her account,*" that is to say, with a meat-offering, the symbol of the fruit of her walk and conduct before Yahweh. Being the sacrificial gift of a wife who had gone aside and was suspected of adultery, this meat-offering could not possess the character of the ordinary meat-offerings, which shadowed forth the fruit of the **sanctification of life in good works**; could not consist, that is to say, of fine wheat flour, but only of barley meal.

Barley was worth only half as much as wheat, so that only the poorer classes, or the people generally in times of great distress, used barley meal as their daily food while those who were better off used it for fodder. Barley meal was prescribed for this sacrifice, neither as a sign that the adulteress had conducted herself like an irrational animal, nor "*because the persons presenting the offering were invoking the punishment of a crime,* *and not the favor of Yahweh*" because the guilt of a woman was not yet established; nor even, taking a milder view of the matter, to indicate that the one offering might be innocent, and in that case no offering at all was required, but to represent the questionable repute in which the woman stood, or the ambiguous, suspicious character of her conduct. Because such conduct as hers did not proceed from the Spirit of Yahweh, and was not carried out in prayer; oil and incense, the symbols of the Spirit of Yahweh and prayer, were not to be added to her offering. It was an offering of jealousy and the object was to bring the ground of that jealousy to light; and in this respect it is called the "*meat-offering of remembrance,*" of the woman before Yahweh, namely, "*the remembrance of iniquity,*" bringing her crime to remembrance before the Lord, that it might be judged by Him.

The course prescribed in this case was that if the suspected wife was innocent, she might not continue under the reproach of her husband's jealousy, and, if guilty, her sin might find her out, and others might hear, fear and take warning.

As I have said and am somewhat repeating; the process of the trial must be that her husband must take her to the priest and desire that she might be put on trial. The Israelites say that the priest was first to endeavor to persuade her to confess the truth, saying like this ...

> *"Dear daughter, perhaps thou was overtaken by drinking wine, or was carried away by the heat of youth or the examples of bad neighbors; come, confess the truth, for the sake of His great name which is described in the most sacred ceremony and do not let it be blotted out with the bitter water."*

If she confessed, saying, "*I am defiled*," she was **not** put to death, but was divorced and lost her dowry; if she said, "*I am pure*," then they proceeded. He must bring an offering of barley-meal, **without oil or FRANKINCENSE**. It is an offering of memorial, to signify that what was to be done was intended as a **religious appeal** to the omniscience and justice of Yahweh. The priest was to prepare the water of jealousy, the **holy water out of the laver** at which the priests were to wash when they ministered; this must be brought in an earthen vessel, containing, *they say*, about a pint; and it must be an earthen vessel, because the coarser and plainer everything was the more agreeable it was to the occasion. Dust must be put into the water, to signify the reproach she lay under, and the shame she ought to take to herself, putting her mouth in the dust; but dust from the floor of the tabernacle, to put an honor upon everything that pertained to the place that Yahweh had chosen to put His name there, and to keep up in the people a reverence for it. The woman was to be set before the Lord, *"at the east gate"* of the temple-court (*say the Israelites*), and her head was to be uncovered, in token of her sorrowful condition; and there she stood for a spectacle to the world, that other women might learn not to do after her lewdness. Only the Israelites say, "*Her own servants were not to be present, that she might not seem vile in their sight, who were to give honor to her; her husband also must be dismissed.*" The priest was to adjure her to tell the truth and to denounce the curse of Yahweh against her if she were guilty and to declare what would be the effect of her drinking the water of jealousy. He must assure her that if she were innocent, the water would do her no harm. None need fear the curse of the Law if they have not broken the commands of the Law. But, if she was guilty, this water would be poison to her; it would make her belly swell and her thigh to rot, and she should be a curse or abomination among her people. To this she must say, Amen, as Israel must do to the curses pronounced on mount Ebal (Deuteronomy 27:15-26). Some think the Amen, ***being doubled***, respects both parts of the adjuration, both that which freed her if innocent and that which condemned her if guilty. No woman, if she were guilty, could say Amen to this adjuration, and drink the water upon it, unless she disbelieved the truth of Yahweh or defied His justice, and had come to such a hard-heartedness in sin as to challenge Yahweh the Almighty to do His worst, and choose rather to venture upon His curse than to give Him glory by making confession; thus has whoredom taken away from the heart. The priest was to write this curse in a scrip or scroll of parchment, **verbatim**—word for word, as he had expressed it, and then to wipe or scrape out what he had written into the water (v-23), to signify that it was that curse which impregnated the water, and gave it its strength to effect what was intended. It signified that, if she was innocent, the curse should be blotted out and never appear against her, as it is written (Isaiah 43:25), "*I am He that blotteth out thy transgression,*" and (Psalms 51:9), "*Blot out my iniquities*". But, if she were guilty, the curse, as it was written, being infused into the water, would enter into her bowels with the water, even like oil into her bones (Psalms 109:18), as we read of a curse entering into a house (Zechariah 5:4). The woman must then drink the water (v-24). It is called the bitter water; some think because they put wormwood in it to make it bitter, or rather because it caused the curse. Thus, sin is called an evil thing and bitter for the same reason, because it causes the curse (Jeremiah 2:19). If she had been guilty (*and otherwise it did not cause the curse*), she was made to know that though her stolen waters had been sweet and her bread eaten in secret and pleasant, yet the end was bitter as wormwood. Let all that meddle with forbidden pleasures know that they will be bitterness in the latter end. **The Israelites say** that if, upon denouncing the curse, the woman was so terrified that she would not drink the water, but confessed that she was defiled, the priest threw down the water, and cast her offering among the ashes, and she was divorced without dowry. If she did not confess and yet would not drink, they forced her to it; and, if she was ready to throw it up again, they hastened her away, that she might not pollute the holy place. Before she drank the water, the jealousy-offering was waved and offered upon the altar. A handful of it was burned for a memorial and the remainder of it was eaten by the priest, **unless the husband was a priest**, and then it was scattered among the ashes. This offering in the midst of the transaction signified that the whole was an appeal to Yahweh, as Yahweh who knows all things and from whom no secret is hid. All things being thus performed according to the Law, they were to wait the issue. The water, with a little dust put into it, and the scrapings of a written parchment, had no natural tendency at all to do either good or bad; but if Yahweh was thus appealed to in the way of an instituted ordinance, though otherwise the innocent might have continued under suspicion and the guilty undiscovered, yet Yahweh would so far own his own institution as that in a little time, by the miraculous operation of Providence, the innocence of the innocent should be cleared, and the sin of the guilty should find them out. If the suspected woman was really guilty, the water she drank would be poison to her; her belly would swell and her thigh rot by a vile disease for vile deserts, and she would mourn at the last when her flesh and body were consumed. Bishop Patrick says, **from some of the Israelite writers**, that the effect of these waters appeared **immediately**; she grew pale and her eyes began to go out of her head. Dr. Lightfoot says that **sometimes it appeared not for two or three years**, but she bore no children, was sickly and rotted at last; it is probable that some indications appeared immediately. **The rabbis say** that the **adulterer** also died in the same day and hour that the adulteress did and in the same manner too, that his belly swelled and his secret parts rotted. A disease perhaps not much unlike that which in those latter ages the avenging hand of a righteous Yahweh had made the scourge of uncleanness and with which whores and whoremongers were infected and ruined one another since they escaped punishment from men. **The Israelite doctors** add that the waters had this effect upon the adulteress only in case the husband had never offended in the same way. Men, knowing their own crimes, were content not to know their wives' crimes. And to this perhaps may refer the threatening (Hosea 4:14), "*I will not punish your spouses when they commit adultery, for you yourselves are separated with whores.*" If she were innocent, the water she drank would be physic to her: "*She shall be free, and shall conceive seed*" (v-28). **The Israelite writers** magnify the good effects of this water to the innocent woman, that, to recompense her for the wrong done to her by the suspicion, she should, after the drinking of those waters, be stronger and look better than ever; if she was sickly, she should become healthful, should bear a man-child, and have easy labor.

FRANKINCENSE OIL: The **health** benefits of **FRANKINCENSE Essential Oil** can be attributed to its properties as an antiseptic, disinfectant, astringent, carminative, cicatrisant, cytophylactic, digestive, diuretic, emenagogue, expectorant, sedative, tonic, uterine and vulnerary substance.

FRANKINCENSE Oil is extracted from the gum or resin from **FRANKINCENSE** or Olibanum trees, whose scientific name is **Boswellia Carteri**. The main components of this essential oil are Alpha Pinene, Actanol, Bornyl Acetate, Linalool, Octyl Acetate, Incensole and Incensyl Acetate. **FRANKINCENSE** has been a popular ingredient in cosmetics and **incense** burners for centuries. It has even been found in the remains of ancient Egyptian and Anglo-Saxon civilizations. Furthermore, it is closely associated with religious traditions and rites, particularly in the believers.

CHAPTER SEVEN

1 CHRONICLES 9:29

This chapter is still dealing with the things of the Israelite tabernacle. Here is the <u>New American Standard Version</u> of this passage ...

> *<u>"Now some of them had charge of the utensils of service, for they counted them when they brought them in and when they took them out. 29 Some of them also were appointed over the furniture and over all the utensils of the sanctuary and over the fine flour and the wine and the oil and the</u>* **FRANKINCENSE** *<u>and the spices. 30 Some of the sons of the priests prepared the mixing of the spices. 31 Mattithiah, one of the Levites, who was the firstborn of Shallum the Korahite, had the responsibility over the things which were baked in pans. 32 Some of their relatives of the sons of the Kohathites were over the showbread to prepare it every sabbath."</u>*

Besides the gatekeepers, some Levites were responsible for the articles and foodstuffs **in the temple service**. This included the furnishings, vessels, flour, wine, oil, incense, spices and bread. Other Levites were musicians who were free from all other duties and for convenience were assigned **living quarters in the temple complex itself**.

As to all of the Israelites, some were set over the vessels in general and over all the holy vessels which were **used for the**

daily sacrificial service, and over the **fine** flour and **incense** (***FRANKINCENSE***) which was required therein for **the meat and drink offerings**, and the spices for the holy **perfumes**.

Everyone knew his charge. Some were entrusted with the ministering vessels, to bring them in and out. Others were appointed to prepare the fine flour, wine, oil, etc.. Others, **that were priests**, made up the holy anointing oil. Others took care of the meat-offerings: Others of the show-bread. As in other great houses, so in Yahweh's house, the work is likely to be done well when everyone knows the duty of his place and makes a business of it. Yahweh is the Yahweh of order.

As far as the **FRANKINCENSE** is concerned, there are many health benefits of **FRANKINCENSE ESSENTIAL OIL**.

Apart from being used as a cosmetic and as a fragrance, **FRANKINCENSE OIL** has numerous **medicinal** uses, which are summarized below.

Immune System: FRANKINCENSE OIL is effective as an **antiseptic**, and even the fumes or smoke obtained from burning it have antiseptic and disinfectant qualities that eliminate the germs in the space where the smoke filters out. It can be applied on wounds without any known side effects to protect them from tetanus and becoming septic. It is equally good on **internal wounds** and protects them from developing infections.

Oral Health: Those same antiseptic qualities also make **FRANKINCENSE OIL** a useful preventative measure against oral issues, like bad breath, toothaches, cavities, mouth sores and other infections. Look for natural oral care products that include **FRANKINCENSE OIL** if you enjoy the flavor or aroma, and want to include a strong antiseptic in your **health** regimen. You can even create your own all-natural toothpaste with **FRANKINCENSE OIL** and baking soda, or a mouthwash with water and peppermint oil.

Astringent: The astringent property of **FRANKINCENSE OIL** has many benefits, because it strengthens gums, hair roots, tones and lifts skin, contracts muscles, intestines and blood vessels, and thereby gives protection from premature losses of teeth and hair. This astringent quality also reduces the appearance of wrinkles, and combats the loss of firmness of intestines, abdominal muscles and limbs associated with age. Above all, **FRANKINCENSE** acts as a coagulant, helping to stop bleeding from wounds and cuts. This astringent property also helps to relieve diarrhea of various types.

CHAPTER EIGHT

NEHEMIAH 13:5&9

This is the New American Standard Version of the above verses ...

> "Now prior to this, Eliashib the priest, who was appointed over the chambers of the house of our Yahweh, being related to Tobiah, 5 had prepared a large room for him, where formerly they put the grain offerings, the **FRANKINCENSE**, the utensils and the tithes of grain, wine and oil prescribed for the Levites, the singers and the gatekeepers, and the contributions for the priests. 6 But during all this time I was not in Jerusalem, for in the thirty-second year of Artaxerxes king of Babylon I had gone to the king. After some time, however, I asked leave from the king, 7 and I came to Jerusalem and learned about the **evil that Eliashib had done for Tobiah**, by preparing a room for him in the courts of the house of Yahweh. 8 **It was very displeasing to me, so I threw all of Tobiah's household goods out of the room.** 9 Then I gave an order and they cleansed the rooms; and I returned there the utensils of the house of Yahweh with the grain offerings and the **FRANKINCENSE**."

You will see that **FRANKINCENSE** was used two times in this paragraph. I will deal first with the verses and then I will speak some more about **FRANKINCENSE**.

Nehemiah came to Jerusalem in the twentieth year of Artaxerxes, and remained there till the thirty-second year,

twelve years; then returned to Babylon and stayed one year; got leave to revisit his brethren; and found matters as stated in this chapter. Nehemiah acted as Jesus did when he found the courts of the Lord's house profaned. He overthrew the tables of the money-changers and the seats of those who sold doves. The expression, *"the offerings of the priests"* is the portion of the offerings assigned for their sustenance to the priests. The expression *"after certain days,"* probably meant at the end of a year which is a meaning that the phrase often has. Nehemiah probably went to the court at Babylon in 433 B.C., and returned to Jerusalem in 432 B.C.. The "*great chamber*" assigned to Tobiah, contained, it would seem, more than one apartment. Artaxerxes is called the king of Babylon because his rule over the Persian Empire included Babylon. Nehemiah then returned to Artaxerxes. Sometime later (*perhaps two years or more*), Nehemiah asked to return to Jerusalem. How long he stayed this **second time is not stated.** Malachi may have ministered about that same time.

Hearing what the high priest had done to Tobiah (*Nehemiah called it an evil thing*), Nehemiah was deeply distressed. Eliashib had been involved in restoring the walls (3:1), but now **inconsistently** he had allowed an opponent to reside **inside the temple complex**! Understandably, Nehemiah was so angry that he went into the temple room and tossed out all of Tobiah's household goods. He then had the **rooms** (*apparently Tobiah* *had also occupied some rooms adjacent to the large chamber)* purified, either ceremonially or by fumigation or both, and restored the temple articles and offerings that belonged there.

Not only were some of the Israelites married to **Ammonites or Moabites**, but also an **Ammonite was living in the Israelite temple**! Tobiah the Ammonite (4:3) had been given a room in the temple by Eliashib the high priest (13:28). Eliashib is the first one named in the list of workers (3:1), and yet **he had become a traitor**. Why? **Because one of his relatives was married to Sanballat's daughter (13:28), and Sanballat and Tobiah were friends. They were all a part of the secret faction in Jerusalem that was fraternizing with the enemy**. Sounds just like the United States of America in our day and time.

Just because a family has been active in the assembly a long time and has helped to build the work, is no sign that each generation will be spiritual, or that any generation will remain spiritual. Children and grandchildren can drift from the faith and try to bluff their way **on the testimony of their ancestors**, and fathers and mothers can depart from the faith just to please their children. **Eliashib's relative was privileged to be born into the priestly family, yet he threw away his future ministry by marrying the wrong woman**; and Eliashib apparently approved of it. Does this sound like the U.S.A. today and getting worse?

All this happened while Nehemiah was away at the palace, which suggests that those he appointed to lead in his absence had failed in their oversight. It does not take long for the enemy to capture leadership, and too often the people will blindly follow their leaders in the path of compromise and disobedience. It was hard enough that an Ammonite was living in the temple (*White House*?), and that an Israelite high priest had let him in; but this intruder was using a room dedicated to Yahweh for the storing of the offerings used by the Levites. He defiled the temple by his presence and robbed the servants of Yahweh at the same time. Nehemiah lost no time throwing out both the man and his furniture, rededicating the room to the Lord, and using it again for its intended purpose. Like our Lord, Nehemiah had to cleanse the temple; and it appears that he had to do it alone.

But, in all that time he was not at Jerusalem. Eliashib had concluded that, as Nehemiah had departed from Jerusalem and, on the expiration of his allotted term of absence, had resigned his government, he had gone not to return and began to use great liberties, and, there being none left whose authority or frown he dreaded, allowed himself to do **things most unworthy of his sacred office**, and which, though in unison with his own **irreligious** character, he would not have dared to attempt during the residence of the pious governor. **Nehemiah resided 12 years as Governor of Jerusalem**, and having succeeded in repairing and re-fortifying the city, he, at the end of that period, returned to his duties in Shushan.

How long he remained there is not expressly said, but "*after certain days*," which is a Scriptural phraseology for a year or a number of years, he obtained leave to **resume the government of Jerusalem**; and, to his deep mortification and regret, found matters in the neglected and disorderly state here described. Such gross irregularities as were practiced - such **extraordinary corruptions** as had crept in -evidently implied the lapse of a considerable time. Besides, they exhibit the character of Eliashib, **the high priest, in a most unfavorable light**; for while he ought, by his office, to have preserved the inviolable sanctity of the temple and its furniture, his influence had been **directly exercised for evil**; especially, he had given permission and countenance to a most indecent outrage - the appropriation of **the best apartments in the sacred building to a pagan governor, one of the worst and most determined enemies of the people and the worship of Yahweh**. At the very first reform, Nehemiah, on his second visit, resolved upon, was the stopping of this gross profanation; and the chamber which had been polluted by the residence of **the idolatrous Ammonite** was, after undergoing the process of ritual purification, restored to its proper use - a storehouse for the sacred vessels. To repeat ...

Eliashib the high priest had given up to his relative, Tobiah the **Ammonite** a large chamber in the temple, i.e., in the fore-court of the temple, probably for his use as a dwelling when he visited Jerusalem. On his return, Nehemiah immediately cast all the furniture of Tobiah out of this chamber, purified the chambers, and restored them to their proper use as a magazine for the temple stores. Eliashib was set over the chambers of the house of Yahweh; for such oversight would certainly be entrusted to **no** simple priest, though this addition shows that this oversight **did not absolutely form part of the high priest's office**. Eliashib, being a relation of Tobiah, prepared him a chamber. How Tobiah was related to Eliashib is nowhere stated. However, he **might** have been **nearly** related to the high priest. His grandson had married Sanballat's daughter.

Nehemiah was informed by the good people who were troubled at what an intimacy had grown between their **chief priest and their chief enemy**, it grieved him sorely that Yahweh's house should be so profaned.

But we need to look at **FRANKINCENSE** some more as it is mentioned in this verse.

EMENAGOGUE: FRANKINCENSE essential oil reduces obstructed and delayed menstruation and delays the advent of menopause. It also helps curing other symptoms associated with menses and

Post Menstrual Syndrome, such as pain in the abdominal region, **nausea, headache, fatigue and mood swings**.

CARMINATIVE: FRANKINCENSE OIL eliminates gas and prevents it from building up in the body. This removal of excess gas from the intestines also gives relief from associated problems like stomach aches, pain in the abdominal region and chest, abnormal amounts of sweating, uneasiness, indigestion and many other related conditions.

CICATRISANT: This is an interesting property of **FRANKINCENSE OIL**, and since skin health and anti-aging are such hot topics these days, this essential oil has become even more important! When applied topically or inhaled, it can make the scars and after marks of boils, acne and pox on the skin fade at a much faster rate. This also includes the fading of **stretch marks, surgery marks, and fat cracks** associated with pregnancy and delivery of children.

DIGESTIVE: Suffering from indigestion due to that turkey last night? A patient of chronic indigestion and acidity? Fed up with those **antacids?** Then you should try **FRANKINCENSE OIL** instead. This oil has **digestive** properties **without any side effects**, and it facilitates digestion the way most **medicines** should, unlike common antacids which only suppress the symptoms. This oil speeds up the secretion of digestive juices (*gastric juices, bile and acids*) in the stomach and facilitates movement of food through the intestines by stimulating peristaltic motion. This means an all-around improvement in the digestion of food.

CHAPTER NINE

SONG OF SOLOMON 3:6

As usual, this is where the afore mentioned verse is in the <u>New American Standard Version</u> that also deals with **FRANKINCENSE** ...

> "**What is this coming up from the wilderness like columns of smoke, perfumed with myrrh and FRANKINCENSE, with all scented powders of the merchant?** 7 "Behold, **it is the traveling couch of Solomon**; sixty mighty men around it, of the mighty men of Israel. 8 "All of them are wielders of the sword, expert in war; each man has his sword at his side, guarding against the terrors of the night. 9 "King Solomon has made for himself a **sedan chair from the timber of Lebanon**. 10 "He made its posts of silver, its back of gold and its seat of purple fabric, with its interior lovingly fitted out by the daughters of Jerusalem. 11 "Go forth, O daughters of Zion, and gaze on King Solomon with the crown with which his mother has crowned him **on the day of his wedding**, and **on the day of his gladness of heart**" [3:6-11].

Going to Egypt was called descending or going down; coming from it was termed **coming up**. The bride, having risen, goes after her spouse to the country, and the clouds of **incense** (**FRANKINCENSE**) arising from her seemed like pillars of smoke; and the appearance was so splendid as to attract the admiration of her own women, who converse about her splendor, excellence, etc., and then take occasion to describe **Solomon's nuptial bed and chariot**. Some think that it is the bridegroom who is spoken of here. With this verse the third night is supposed to end. These were the guards about the pavilion of the bridegroom, who were placed there because of fear in the **night**. The security and state of the prince required such a guard as this, and the **passage is to be literally understood**. They were swordsmen. Every man had a sword, and was well instructed how to use it. The superb piece of embroidery, wrought by some of the noble maids of Jerusalem, and, as a proof of their affection, respect and love, presented to the **bride and bridegroom, on their nuptial day**.

The couch is made of wooden lattices painted and gilded. The inside is painted with baskets of flowers, intermixed with little mottoes according to the fancy of the artist. Solomon's couch may have been of the same kind, and decorated in the same way; and the **paving with love** may refer to the verses worked either on the hangings or embroidered carpet. And as this was **done by the daughters of Jerusalem**, they might have expressed the most striking parts of such a chaste history of love.

This is the exhortation of the companions of the bride to the females of the city to examine the superb appearance of the bridegroom, and especially the nuptial crown, which appears to have been made by Bathsheba, who it is supposed **might have**

lived until the time of Solomon's marriage with the daughter of Pharaoh. It is conjectured that the prophet referred to a nuptial crown. But a crown, both on the bride and bridegroom, was common among most people on such occasions. This was the day in which all his wishes were crowned, by being united to that female whom beyond all others he loved.

Pillars of smoke here is an image of delight and pleasure. **FRANKINCENSE** and other perfumes are burned in such abundance round the bridal procession that the whole procession appears from the distance to be one of moving wreaths and columns of smoke. The pomp and beauty of this bridal procession is wholly appropriate in light of the event's significance. The Scriptures teach that marriage is one of the most important events in a person's life. Therefore it is fitting that the union of a couple be commemorated in a special way. The current practice of couples casually living together apart from the bonds of marriage demonstrates how unfashionable genuine commitment to another person has become in contemporary society.

The sixty warriors accompanying the carriage were friends of the groom. It was common for a groom's friends to go with him in the wedding procession. But they were also the noblest and **most experienced soldiers in Israel**, probably **Solomon's royal bodyguard**. David had a bodyguard and so **possibly** did Solomon.

Since the caravan may have had to travel some distance, the king was taking no chances with the safety of his bride. If bandits would appear at **night** and terrorize the bride, the soldiers were ready for them. **The lesson is valid today** for a would-be husband. He should give proper thought and planning to protect his bride. In one form, this takes providing economic security for her.

At last the day arrived for the Shulamite to wed her beloved! Not only would he claim her as his wife, but she would discover that her husband **was the king**! The glorious procession appears on the horizon. It is Solomon's bride being carried in her richly decorated palanquin, surrounded by sixty of Solomon's bravest soldiers, with a cloud of fragrant **incense (FRANKINCENSE)** above her. She wears a wedding crown given to her by Solomon's mother. The daughters of Jerusalem get excited and sing to each other, "*Go forth, O daughters of Zion!*" The bride has her attendants, the king has joy in his heart, and the time has finally come for the wedding to take place.

In modern marriages, the bride is the center of attention, and "*What did the bride wear?*" is the big question. But the king is more concerned with her beauty than with her attire. He has claimed her for himself and it is now their wedding night. In all cases in the Bible, the bride always comes to Yahweh. Tonight she will take her hair down as a symbol that she belongs to him and she has nothing to hide. His speech opens and closes with, "*You are beautiful!*" The images the king uses to describe her beauty may seem strange to us, but measures of beauty change from age to age and culture to culture.

The doves' eyes would reflect peace and depth. The bride's teeth were clean, even and beautiful. When you remember that ancient peoples did not quite understand dental hygiene, this is an admirable trait. Healthy teeth would also affect her breath (7:8). She had a queenly neck and a posture with it that showed control, power and stability. She was a tower of strength! The "*mountains of **myrrh***" refer to her breasts, which he would enjoy all night until the dawn would break, and she would also enjoy his expressions of love.

Beginning in verse 8, six times he calls her his "*spouse*" or his bride. After the marriage is consummated, she is no longer a bride but a wife. They are enjoying a "*mountaintop experience*" as they share their love and he tells her how beautiful she is. "*Thy love*" in verse 10 refers to her words and actions and not just her feelings. It could be translated "*love-making.*" He rejoices that **his bride is a virgin**, "*a garden locked up, a spring enclosed and a fountain sealed*" (v-12). This is another evidence that the Lord wants both the man and the woman to stay sexually pure. Conjugal love is pictured in terms of satisfying thirst (v-15) and exploring a beautiful and fruitful garden that

never grows old. The bride is the garden and the bridegroom prays that the winds of life will make her even more beautiful and desirable. We may not appreciate the north wind, but even it can help us mature in our love. With this lovely preparation completed, the bride is now ready, and she invites her husband to come into his garden and drink the living water and eat the nourishing fruits. He accepts her loving invitation and then says, "*I have come into my garden*!" They had feasted at the beginning of their relationship (1:2-2:7), but it was nothing like this! They now had truly tasted the fruits and enjoyed the wine, milk and fragrant spices.

Who speaks in verse 5? Is it the bride telling her husband-lover that he may visit the garden often? "*Drink deeply*" ("*drink your fill*") suggests that there is always more to learn and enjoy as the marriage progresses. But the noun "*beloved*" is plural and can be translated "*lovers*." Surely the **daughters of Jerusalem** are not there at that private sacred moment! It has been suggested that this may be Yahweh speaking to the couple and through them encouraging all married couples to enjoy the blessings of married love, for He created sex for pleasure as well as for procreation.

It seems true that it is a **woman** that is being brought forward to those who ask, even if she is yet too far off to be seen by them, because they recognize in the festal gorgeous procession a marriage party. That the company comes up from the wilderness, it may be through the wilderness which separates Jerusalem from Jericho, is in accordance with the fact that a **maiden from Galilee** is being brought up, and that the procession has taken the way through the Jordan valley; but the scene has also a typical coloring; for the wilderness is, since the time of the Mosaic deliverance out of Egypt, an emblem of the transition from a state of bondage to freedom, from humiliation to glory. The pomp is like that of a procession before which the censer of **FRANKINCENSE** is swung. Columns of smoke from the burning **incense** mark the line of the procession before and after. I will note that the circumstance of the Tôra required **myrrh** as a component part **of the holy oil** (Exodus 30:23), and **FRANKINCENSE** as a component **part of the holy incense** (Exodus 30:34), and points to Arabia as the source whence they were obtained.

The daughters of Jerusalem, to whom the charge was given, had looked upon the bride because she was **black** (ch. 1:6); but now they admire her, and speak of her with great respect. Who is this? How beautiful she looks! Who would have expected such a comely and magnificent person **to come out of the wilderness**?

This is applicable to the Israelite assembly, when, after forty years' wandering in the wilderness, they came out of it, to take a glorious possession of the land of promise; and this may very well be illustrated by what Balaam said of them at that time, when they ascended out of the *"wilderness like pillars of smoke, and he stood admiring them: From the top of the rocks I see him. How goodly are thy tents, O Jacob"*!

FRANKINCENSE Oil is also very good to use – internally and externally.

Anti-Aging: As a Cytophylactic, **FRANKINCENSE OIL** promotes regeneration of **healthy cells** and also keeps the existing cells and tissues healthy. When you combine this aspect of **FRANKINCENSE OIL** with its powerful astringent capabilities, you have a potent anti-aging quality for **FRANKINCENSE OIL** that is often used. It can help you to **eliminate sun spots, remove micro-wrinkles around the eyes and cheeks, and generally tone and tighten skin all over your body, while simultaneously replacing old or dying cells with new, healthy ones**!

Tonic: Overall, **FRANKINCENSE** essential oil tones and boosts **health** and is therefore considered a tonic. It benefits all the systems operating in the body, including the **respiratory, digestive, nervous and excretory systems**, while also increasing strength by aiding the absorption of nutrients into the body. Furthermore, **FRANKINCENSE OIL strengthens the immune system** and keeps you strong and protected for the future.

<u>Diuretic:</u> If you thought that Lasix and its variants were the only drugs that could help you release water from the body through urination, you were incorrect. Those pharmaceutical options may be instantaneous, but not very safe. **FRANKINCENSE ESSENTIAL OIL** is a natural and safe alternative. **<u>It promotes urination</u>** and helps you lose that extra water weight, as well as **<u>fats, sodium, uric acid and various other toxins</u>** from the body, with the added advantage of **<u>lowering blood pressure</u>**. The best part about this is that **<u>FRANKINCENSE</u>** essential oil is **<u>completely safe and has no adverse side effects.</u>**

The brides eyes, hair, teeth, lips, temples, neck and breasts - to each of these is attached a comparison from nature. The resemblances consist **<u>not so much in outward likeness</u>**, as in the combined sensations of delight produced by contemplating these natural objects. This might be a figure of speech about Jesus getting to "*the mountain of **myrrh** and the hill of **FRANKINCENSE**,*" and also expresses Yahweh taking His abode in His temple on the holy hill of Zion, where **<u>FRANKINCENSE</u>** was offered **<u>until the spiritual day-break at the first advent of Messiah</u>** about 4 B.C.. It seems as if the Israelite bride was deeply veiled.

CHAPTER TEN

SONG OF SOLOMON 4:6

This chapter has the word **FRANKINCENSE** listed twice. Here is the first part, which continues in the next part which we use under the next chapter ...

*"How beautiful you are, my darling, how beautiful you are! Your eyes are like doves behind your veil; your hair is like a flock of goats that have descended from Mount Gilead. 2 "Your teeth are like a flock of newly shorn ewes which have come up from their washing, all of which bear twins, and not one among them has lost her young. 3 "Your lips are like a scarlet thread, and your mouth is lovely. Your temples are like a slice of a pomegranate behind your veil. 4 "Your neck is like the tower of David, built with rows of stones on which are hung a thousand shields, all the round shields of the mighty men. "Your two breasts are like two fawns, twins of a gazelle which feed among the lilies. 6 "Until the cool of the day when the shadows flee away, I will go my way to the mountain of **myrrh** and to the hill of* **FRANKINCENSE**."

This **figurative language** is probably the same as the mountains of Bether (Song of Solomon 2:17), the mountains where the **trees** grew from which **myrrh** and **incense** was extracted. It appears that this is about **the bride's entry into the city of David, and her marriage there with the king. Israelite interpreters** regard this part of the poem as symbolizing the "*first*" entrance of the assembly of the *"old testament"* into the land of promise, and her spiritual espousals, and communion with the King of kings, through the erection of Solomon's Temple and the institution of its acceptable worship.

The first to speak on their wedding night was Solomon and his words praised his bride's beauty. Three times on the wedding night he told her that she was beautiful. When the groom said his bride's breasts were like fawns, he was comparing **their softness**, not their color or form. Looking on the soft coat of a little fawn makes a person want to stroke it. Solomon wanted his bride to know that her soft and gentle beauty had kindled his desire for her and he wished to express that desire with his caresses. Solomon was overcome with desire for his bride and resolved to fulfill her silent request. The mountain of **myrrh** and the hill of **incense** (***FRANKINCENSE***) refer to the beloved's breasts. The primary point of comparison was not in the visual area, but rather in the **realms of function and value. Myrrh and incense** were used to perfume the body as well as the bedroom in order to make a person and the surroundings more attractive. They would give their love to each other till the morning. A **mountain** of **myrrh** or a **hill** of **FRANKINCENSE** would have been greatly valued. **To Solomon, therefore, his bride's breasts were attractive and of great value to him**. The breasts are compared to a twin pair of young gazelles in respect of their equality and youthful freshness, and the bosom on which they raise themselves is compared to a meadow covered with lilies, on which the twin-pair of young gazelles feed. With this tender lovely image the praise of the attractions of the chosen one is interrupted. If one counts the lips and the mouth as a part of the body, which they surely are, there are seven things here praised, as some rightly counts (the eyes, the hair, teeth, mouth, temples, neck and breasts); and others speak rightly of the **sevenfold beauty of the bride**.

As we continue, we will look again at **FRANKINCENSE** as we have done from the beginning of my book.

RESPIRATORY ISSUES: It soothes coughs and eliminates phlegm deposited in the respiratory tracts and the lungs. **FRANKINCENSE ESSENTIAL OILS** also provides relief from bronchitis and congestion of nasal tract, larynx, pharynx, bronchi and lungs. Its antidepressant and anti-inflammatory properties also help relax the breathing passages, which can reduce the dangers of asthma attacks, and its antiseptic qualities are what give it the reputation of being an immune system booster! It also eases body pain, headaches, toothaches and balances the rise in body temperature commonly associated with colds.

FRANKINCENSE STRESS & ANXIETY: FRANKINCENSE OIL is very effective as a **sedative**, because it induces a feeling of mental peace, relaxation, satisfaction and spirituality. It also awakens insight, makes you more introspective and lowers anxiety, anger and stress. When feeling anxious or if you anticipate some sort of stressful episode, add some **FRANKINCENSE OIL** to a diffuser or a vaporizer. **FRANKINCENSE ESSENTIAL OIL** promotes deep breathing and relaxation, which can open your breathing passages and reduce blood pressure, moving your mental state back to calmness.

UTERINE: This oil is very good for uterine health. Since it regulates the production of the **estrogen hormone**, it reduces the chances of post-menopause tumor or cyst formation in the uterus, also known as **uterine cancer**. In terms of the pre-menopause period, it keeps a woman's uterus healthy by regulating proper menstrual cycles. It also **treats or regulates gynecologic conditions** or stressors that can lead to complicated dysfunctions in certain women.

CHAPTER ELEVEN

SONG OF SOLOMON 4:14

This chapter has one more verse that speaks of **FRANKINCENSE** which is quoted now from the <u>New American Standard Version</u> ...

> *"<u>Nard and saffron, calamus and cinnamon, with all the trees of</u> <u>**FRANKINCENSE**, **Myrrh** and aloes, along with all the finest spices."</u>*

This continues with the **fairness** or **beauty** of the maiden listed in the entire chapter. I do not have the time and space in this book to deal with all these things, one at a time, that are listed in this chapter, so I will take here only the one verse that is mentioned.

<u>Seven kinds of spices</u> (*some of them with **Indian** names, e.g. aloes, spikenard, saffron*) are enumerated as found in this **<u>symbolic garden</u>**. They are for the most part, pure exotics which have formed for **<u>countless ages</u>**, articles of commerce in the East, and were brought at that time in Solomon's ships from southern Arabia, the great Indian Peninsula, and perhaps the islands of the Indian Archipelago. The picture here is best regarded as a purely ideal one, having no corresponding reality but in the **bride** herself. The beauties and attractions of both north and south of Lebanon with its **<u>streams of sparkling water</u>**

and fresh mountain air, of Engedi with its tropical climate and henna plantations, of the spice-groves of Arabia Felix, and of the rarest products of the distant mysterious Ophir - **all combine to furnish one glorious representation, "Thou art all fair!"**

By extending the **metaphor of the garden**, Solomon conveyed to his beloved how much he valued her purity. She was like a rich exotic garden, with rare and valuable plant life. Such a garden was therefore valuable, attractive and desirable. Included were fruits, flowers, plants, trees and spices. Pomegranates were a delicacy in Bible times. Henna is a flower with white blossoms. **Nard is a fragrant ointment from a plant native to India**.

As "*nards*" refer to **varieties** of the nard, perhaps to the Indian and the Jamanic spoken of by Strabo and others, so "***all kinds** of incense trees*" refers definitely to the Indian-Arab **varieties of the incense tree** and its fragrant resin; it has its name from the white and transparent seeds of its resin. Thus, **FRANKINCENSE** is a word derived from the Pheonicians. Saffron is a powder from the pistils of a plant in the crocus family. Calamus is possibly **sweet cane** which is an ingredient in the "*holy anointing oil*" for the high priest. These ointments are associated with Jesus' death, as well as with Israelites' feasts. Other perfumes were cinnamon, from the bark of a tall tree, **myrrh** and aloes, a plant native to an island in the Red Sea, whose partially decayed wood gives off a fragrance. Those items would make an unusual garden, valuable for its pleasant tastes, sights and smells. Similarly, **Solomon valued his bride for her pleasing attractiveness**.

Solomon pictures this figurative garden as a pleasant garden. And well may a very great delight be compared to the delight taken in a garden, when the happiness of **Solomon** is happy with his bride. It can look back to **Adam** when innocency was represented by the putting of him into a garden, a garden of pleasure, the garden in Eden. The Israelite assembly is fitly compared to a garden, to a garden which, as was usual, had a fountain in it. Where Solomon made himself gardens and orchards, he made himself pools of water, not only for curiosity and diversion, but for use to water the garden. Eden was well watered. It is a garden **enclosed**, a paradise separated from the common earth. It is appropriated to Yahweh; He has set it apart for Himself; Israel was Yahweh's portion, the lot of His inheritance. It is enclosed for secrecy; the saints were Yahweh's hidden ones, therefore the world knows them not; Jesus walks in his garden unseen. It is enclosed for safety; a hedge of protection is made about it, which all the powers of darkness cannot either find or make a gap in. Yahweh's vineyard is fenced (Isaiah 5:2); there is a wall about it, **a wall of fire**. It has a spring in it, and a fountain, but it is a spring shut up and a fountain sealed, which sends its streams abroad, but is itself carefully locked up, that it may not by any injurious hand be muddied or polluted. The believers are as gardens enclosed; **grace in them** is as a spring shut up there in the hidden man of the heart, where the water that Jesus gives is a well of living water. The *"old-testament"* Israelite assembly was a garden enclosed by the partition wall of the ceremonial law. The Bible was then a spring shut up and a fountain sealed; **it was confined to one nation**; but now the wall of separation is removed, the good news is preached to every nation and in Jesus there is neither Greek nor Israelite. It is as the Garden of Eden, where the Lord Yahweh made to grow every tree that is pleasant to the sight and good for food. Yahweh's plants, or plantations, are an orchard of pomegranates with pleasant fruits. It is not like the vineyard of the man void of understanding that was grown over with thorns and thistles; but here are fruits, pleasant fruits, **all trees of FRANKINCENSE, and all the chief spices**. Here are plenty of fruits and great variety, nothing wanting which might either beautify or enrich this garden, might make it either delightful or serviceable to its great Lord. Everything here is the best of its kind. Their chief spices were much more valuable, because they were much more durable than the choicest of our flowers. Solomon was a great master in botany as well as other parts of natural philosophy; he treated largely of trees and perhaps had reference to some specific qualities of the fruits here specified which made them very fit for the purpose for which he alludes to them. But we must be content to observe, in general, the graces in the saints, are very fitly compared to those fruits and spices. They were planted and did not grow of themselves; the trees of righteousness are the planting of the Lord (Isaiah 61:3); grace springs from an incorruptible seed. They are precious and of high value; hence we read of the precious sons of Zion and their precious faith; they are plants of renown. They are pleasant and of a sweet savor to Yahweh and man, and as strong aromatics, diffuse their fragrancy. They are profitable and of great use. Saints are the blessings of this earth, and their graces are their riches, with which they trade as the merchants of the east with their spices. They are permanent and will be preserved to good purpose, when flowers are withered and good for nothing. **Grace, ripened into glory, will last forever**.

Now that we understand what this verse means; let is return to the purpose of my book – **FRANKINCENSE** (again).

VULNERARY: Simply apply a diluted solution of this oil on wounds, or use it blended with a skin cream, and your wounds will **heal faster and be protected from infections**. This oil is equally beneficial in healing internal wounds, cuts and ulcers.

OTHER BENEFITS: It relieves **pain** associated with **rheumatism and arthritis**. It helps heal boils, infected wounds, acne, circulatory problems, **insomnia** and various types of inflammation.

A FEW WORDS OF CAUTION: There are no known adverse side effects. That being said, **FRANKINCENSE** essential oil **should not be used during pregnancy**, since it does act as an emenagogue and astringent.

BLENDING: FRANKINCENSE Oil **blends well** with Lime, Lemon, Orange and other Citrus oils as well as Benzoin, Bergamot, Lavender, **Myrrh**, Pine and Sandalwood oil. This makes it a popular element of many herbalists for various aromatherapy combinations.

CHAPTER TWELVE

ISAIAH 60:6

This is the next to the last verse in the Bible that uses the word **FRANKINCENSE**. The following verse comes from the <u>New American Standard Version</u> from the verse that heads this chapter. The entire context (*which I shall quote*) concerns the glorified **Zion of Israel** ...

*"Arise, shine; for your light has come, and the glory of the Lord has risen upon you. 2 "For behold, darkness will cover the earth and deep darkness the peoples; but the Lord will rise upon you and His glory will appear upon you. 3 "Nations will come to your light, and kings to the brightness of your rising. 4 "Lift up your eyes round about and see; they all gather together, they come to you. Your sons will come from afar, and your daughters will be carried in the arms. 5 "Then you will see and be radiant, and your heart will thrill and rejoice; because the abundance of the sea will be turned to you, the wealth of the nations will come to you. 6 "**A multitude of camels will cover you, the young camels of Midian and Ephah; all those from Sheba will come; they will bring gold and FRANKINCENSE, and will bear good news of the praises of the Lord.** 7 "All the flocks of Kedar will be gathered together to you, the rams of Nebaioth will minister to you; they will go up with acceptance on My altar, and I shall glorify My glorious house. 8 "Who are these who fly like a cloud and like the doves to their lattices? 9 "Surely the coastlands will wait for Me; and the ships of Tarshish will come first, to bring your sons from*

afar, their silver and their gold with them, for the name of the Lord your Yahweh, and for the Holy One of Israel because He has glorified you."

The expression *"shall cover thee"* is speaking of something that shall come in such **multitudes** as to fill one, and to be spread out all over one. Thus we speak of a land being covered with flocks and herds. If you ever go to New Zealand, as you are over the land-scape, you will very seldom see people but you will see multitudes of sheep! Really. I think there are four million people there but I have heard that there are four hundred million sheep. Maybe that will help you to understand what **multitudes** mean in the verse. Thus we speak of a land being covered with flocks, herds and camels. Camels were everywhere and would travel as fast in one day that horses would travel in eight or ten days. They were called *"the ship of the desert."* These fleet animals were so valuable to the inhabitants of Arabia, that they would come bringing their merchandise for the service of the assembly of Yahweh; that is, the wealth of Midian and Ephah would be devoted to Him. One thing needs to be noted. Dromedaries have only one hump on top but camels have two. It is the camels that are noted for their swiftness.

Midian was the fourth son of Abraham and Keturah and was the **father of the Midianites**. The Midianites are frequently mentioned in the Scriptures. As early as the time of Jacob, they were employed in traffic and were associated with the

Ishmaelites in this business, for it was to a company of these people that Joseph was sold by his brethren. The original and appropriate district of the Midianites seems to have been on the east side of the Elanitic branch of the Red Sea, where the Arabian geographers place the city of Madian. But they appear to have spread themselves northward, probably along the desert coast of Mount Seir, to the vicinity of the Moabites; and on the other side, also, they covered a territory extending to the neighborhood of Mount Sinai. Generally, the names Midianites and Ishmaelites seem to have been **nearly** synonymous. **Sheba** is celebrated in the Scriptures chiefly as the place from where the Queen of that country came to visit Solomon. That it abounded in wealth, may be **inferred** from the train which accompanied her, and from the presents with which she gave to Solomon …

*"Now when the queen of Sheba heard about the fame of Solomon concerning the name of the Lord, she came to test him with difficult questions. 2 So she came to Jerusalem **with a very large retinue, with camels carrying spices and very much gold and precious stones.** When she came to Solomon, she spoke with him about all that was in her heart. 3 Solomon answered all her questions; nothing was hidden from the king which he did not explain to her. 4 When the queen of Sheba perceived all the wisdom of Solomon, the house that he had built, 5 the food of his table, the seating of his servants, the attendance of his waiters and their attire, his cupbearers, and his stairway by which he went up to the house of the Lord, there was no more spirit in her. 6 Then she said to the king, "It was a true report which I heard in my own land about your words and your wisdom. 7*

*"Nevertheless I did not believe the reports, until I came and my eyes had seen it. And **behold, the half was not told me**. You exceed in wisdom and prosperity the report which I heard. 8 "How blessed are your men, how blessed are these your servants who stand before you continually and hear your wisdom. 9 "Blessed be the Lord your Yahweh who delighted in you to set you on the **throne of Israel**; because the Lord loved Israel forever, therefore He made you king, to do justice and righteousness." 10 **She gave the king a hundred and twenty talents of gold, and a very great amount of spices and precious stones. Never again did such abundance of spices come in as that which the queen of Sheba gave King Solomon**. 11 Also the ships of Hiram, which brought gold from Ophir, brought in from Ophir a very great number of almug trees and precious stones. 12 The king made of the almug trees supports for the house of the Lord and for the king's house, also lyres and harps for the singers; such almug trees have not come in again nor have they been seen to this day. 13 King Solomon gave to the queen of Sheba all her desire which she requested, besides what he gave her according to his royal bounty. Then she turned and went to her own land together with her servants"* [Kings 10:1-14].

It would be quite wrong to follow a couple of men and draw the conclusion from such prophecies as these, that animal sacrifices will be revived again. **The sacrifice of animals has been abolished once for all by the self-sacrifice of the "Servant of Yahweh;" and by the spiritual revolution which Christianity, i.e., the Messianic religion, as produced**, so far as the consciousness of modern times is concerned, even in Israel itself, it was once for all condemned. **The prophet, indeed, cannot** describe even what belongs to the *"new testament"* in any other than *"old testament"* **colors, because he is still within the *"old testament"* limits**. But from the standpoint of the *"new testament"* fulfilment, that which was merely educational and preparatory, and of which **there will be no revival**, is naturally transformed into the truly essential purpose at which the former aimed.

INCENSE and FRANKINCENSE: They are used almost equally in the Bible. Hebrew is usually *"qetoret,"* once applied to the "*fat*" of rams, the part always burned in sacrifice; once *"qitter,"* marginal, both from the Hebrew, to "*smoke;*" sometimes *"lebona,"* **FRANKINCENSE** (Isaiah 60:6; <u>NIV</u>, "*incense*" *in both passages*), an aromatic compound that gives forth its perfume in burning. Its most general use in Scripture is that perfume that was burned upon the **Israelite altar of incense**. Among both the Hebrews and Egyptians we find no other trace of **incense** than in its sacerdotal use, but in Persian sculptures we see it burned before the king.

MATERIAL: The **incense** employed in the service of the Tabernacle was called "***incense*** *of the aroma*, the ingredients of which are given in Exodus 30:34-35. These consisted of: (1) **stacte**, i.e., '*not the juice squeezed from the highly fragrant* **myrrh** *tree, but probably a species of gum storax resembling* **myrrh**';" (2) **onycha** (literally, a "*scale*"), the shell of the perfumed mollusk, found in the Mediterranean and Red seas and yielding a musky odor when burned; (3) **galbanum** (literally, "*fat*"), a gum that is obtained by making incisions in the bark of a shrub growing in Syria, Arabia and Abyssinia; and (4) **pure FRANKINCENSE** (literally, "*white*"), a pale yellow, semitransparent, pungent resin, which, when burned, is fragrant; it is grown in Arabia and Judea.

PREPARATION: The KJV says "*of each there shall be a like weight,*" i.e., equal parts of the various ingredients, but others think that the meaning is that each ingredient was, in the first place, to be pounded by itself, and then mixed with the rest, for it is possible that the ingredients were not all pounded to the same extent. Besides, it was to be salted (KJV, "*tempered*"), was to be "*pure, and holy,*" i.e., unadulterated with any foreign substance, and was to be reserved exclusively for sacred use, any other application of it being forbidden on pain of being "*cut off from [one's] people.*"

SACRED USE: The person selected to burn **incense** upon the altar of **incense** was Aaron, but in the daily service of the **second Temple**, the office devolved upon the inferior priests, from among whom one was chosen by lot. King Uzziah was punished for presuming to infringe upon this prerogative of the priests. The times of offering **incense** were in the morning, at the time of trimming the lamps, and in the evening, when the lamps were lighted (Exodus 30:7-8). On the Day of Atonement the high priest offered the **incense**.

FIGURATIVE: **Incense** in Scripture is the symbol of prayer; "*May my prayer be counted as **incense** before Thee*." In Revelation 5:8; we meet with the same idea. But ...

> "*It is not prayer alone that is expressed by **incense**. A good or evil savor was to Israel the symbol of a good or godless life; and when, therefore, the sanctuary of Yahweh was kept continually filled with fragrance, they beheld in this the sweet savor, not of prayer alone, but of that life to which, as a priestly nation, they were called*" (W. Milligan, Bib. Ed., 3:226).

CHAPTER THIRTEEN

<u>JEREMIAH 6:20</u>

I will **conclude** with **all** of the passages in the Bible, which is 15, with the passage listed above from the <u>New American Standard Version</u> ...

> *"Thus says the Lord, "Stand by the ways and see and **ask for the ancient paths, where the good way is, and walk in it; and you will find rest for your souls.** But they said, **'We will not walk in it.'** 17 "And I set watchmen over you, saying, 'Listen to the sound of the trumpet!' But they said, **'We will not listen.'** 18 "Therefore hear, O nations, and know, O congregation, what is among them. 19 "Hear, O earth: behold, **I am bringing disaster on this people**, the fruit of their plans, because they have not listened to My words, and as for My law, they have rejected it also. 20 "For what purpose does FRANKINCENSE come to Me from Sheba and the **sweet cane** from a distant land? **Your burnt offerings are not acceptable and your sacrifices are not pleasing to Me**"* [Jeremiah 6:16-20].

The underlined things above were so very important to the Israelites that Yahweh was going to destroy them because they would not listen nor obey His directions. Yahweh had sent prophets (*watchmen*) to warn them.

Ask for the paths that the patriarchs travelled in before you; Abraham, Isaac and Jacob; and, as the Israelites hoped to inherit the promises made to them, tread in their steps.

Let us observe the **metaphor**. A traveler is going to a particular city; he comes to a place where the road divides into several paths, he is afraid of going astray; he stops short, - endeavors to find the right path; he cannot fix his choice. At last he sees another traveler; he inquires of him, gets proper directions - proceeds on his journey - arrives at the desired place - and reposes after his fatigue. The soul needs rest; it can only find this by walking in the good way. The good way is that which had been trodden by the saints from the beginning; it is the old way, the way of faith and holiness. **BELIEVE, LOVE, OBEY; be holy, and be happy**. This is the way; let us inquire for it, and walk in it. But those bad people said, "*We will not walk in it.*" Then they took another way, walked over the precipice, and fell into the bottomless pit; where, instead of rest, they found – a fiery deluge, fed with ever-burning Sulphur - consumed.

Incense (***FRANKINCENSE***) came from Sheba. Sheba was in Arabia, famous for the best **incense**. It was situated toward the southern extremity of the peninsula of Arabia; and was, in respect of Judea, a far country. The **sweet cane**, when dried and pulverized, yields a very fine aromatic smell. This was employed in making the holy anointing oil.

The watchmen were the prophets (Isaiah 52:8). The sound of the trumpet was the signal for flight. Similarly, the prophet's warning was to move men to escape from Yahweh's judgments. Yahweh summons three witnesses to hear His sentence - the ~~Gentiles~~ or better yet, the **nations**, all mankind, Israelites and nations and nature. What does Yahweh do to them, what happens? "*Know what great things I will do to them*." The fathers understood this to be the decree rejecting the Israelites from being the one body of Jesus. The rejection of their **ritual observances** is proclaimed by the two prophets, Isaiah and Jeremiah, who chiefly assisted the two pious kings, Hezekiah and Josiah, in restoring the temple-service. Yahweh rejected not the ceremonial service, but the **substitution** of it for personal holiness and morality.

Judah was in danger of destruction because she had strayed from the ancient paths of Yahweh's righteousness. Yet though Yahweh urged her to walk in the good way where she would find rest, Judah refused. Prophets were like watchmen (*men assigned to watch for and warn a city of impending danger*), but the nation refused to listen.

Judah rejected Yahweh's Law, thinking she could substitute rituals for obedience. Yahweh responded by showing His disdain for **incense** (***FRANKINCENSE***) that had been imported from Sheba in southwest Arabia and for sweet calamus which was probably sweet cane, from a distant land. The elaborate burnt offerings and sacrifices, divorced from a genuine love for Yahweh, did not please Him. Instead of accepting this hypocritical worship, Yahweh vowed to put obstacles in the way of the people so they would stumble. The nature of the obstacles is not given, but it is likely that Yahweh was again referring to the Babylonians.

Were the Israelites guilty? Yes! Did they deserve this punishment? Yes! In fact, Yahweh called the nations and **the earth to bear witness** that He had done all He could to spare them this judgment. They **would not** walk on His path and they **would not** listen to His prophets. Nevertheless, they continued to bring Him their hypocritical worship! Yahweh gave them the right way, but they rejected it. There could be no escape. The Babylonian army would be a formidable obstacle to any-body trying to flee the wrath of Yahweh. The daughter of Zion could not escape. No external services were accepted by Yahweh without obedience of the heart and life, *"Your sweet cane is **not** sweet to me."*

Yahweh had marked out for them the way of salvation in the history of the ancient times. Indeed this very passage teaches that the everlasting ways are the right ones, from which through idolatry the Israelites had wandered into unbeaten paths. It has been said ...

> *"Look inquiringly backwards to ancient history (Deuteronomy 32:7), and see how success and enduring prosperity forsook your fathers when they left the way prescribed to them by Yahweh, to walk in the ways of the heathen (18:15); learn that there is but one way, the way of the fear of Yahweh, on which blessing and salvation are to be found."*

Yahweh rejected their plea, by which they insisted upon their external services as sufficient to atone for all their sins. Alas! It was a frivolous plea (v-20) ...

> *"To what purpose come there to me **incense** and sweet cane, to be burnt for a perfume on the golden altar, though it was the best of the kind, and far-fetched? What care I for your burnt-offerings and your sacrifices?"*

They not only cannot profit Yahweh (*no sacrifice does*, Psalms 50:9), but they do not please Him, for none does this but the sacrifice of the upright; that of the wicked is an abomination to Him. **Sacrifice and incense** were appointed to excite their repentance. Where this good use was made of them, they were acceptable. Yahweh had respect to them and to those that offered them. But when they offered with an **opinion** that thereby they made Yahweh their debtor, and purchased a license to go on in sin, they were so far from being pleasing to Yahweh that they were a provocation to Him. We will go again, as usual, to more on the study of ...

FRANKINCENSE: Is a vegetable resin; brittle, glittering and of a bitter taste, used for the purpose of sacrificial fumigation [Exodus 30:34-36]. It was called **frank** because of the freeness with which, when burned, it gives forth its odor. It burns for a long time, with a steady flame. It is obtained by successive incisions in the bark of a tree called Arbor thuris. The first incision yields the purest and whitest resin, while the product of the after incisions is spotted with yellow, and loses its whiteness altogether as it becomes old. The Hebrews imported their **FRANKINCENSE** from Arabia; but it is remarkable that at present the Arabian olibanum is a very inferior kind, and that the finest **FRANKINCENSE** imported into Turkey comes through Arabia from the islands of the Indian Archipelago. There can be little doubt that the tree which produces the **Indian FRANKINCENSE** is the **Boswellia** serrata of Roxburgh, or Boswellia thurifera of Colebrooke, and bears some resemblance when young to the mountain ash. **It grows to be forty feet high**.

We began this study of the **FRANKINCENSE** and **myrrh** that was given to Jesus at his birth and in every one of the 15 verses we spent some time on **FRANKINCENSE**. It is my opinion that the **FRANKINCENSE** was given to Jesus as a **health product**, very expensive, by the wise men of the East. Reread the ending part of each verse to know all of the things that **FRANKINCENSE** is good for - **HEALTH-WISE!!**

We will now look at the other gift that the Maji gave to Jesus –
<u>MYRRH!!</u>

MYRRH

CHAPTER FOURTEEN

MYRRH

It is very odd that there are fifteen times (same number as **FRANKINCENSE**) that **MYRRH** is mentioned in the Bible but not in the same verses that **FRANKINCENSE** occurs. We will begin with the verses in which both occur in the *"new testament"* about the birth of Jesus and the visit of the wise men and their gifts as we did in the first section. Follow along now ...

> *"Then Herod secretly called the magi and determined from them the exact time the star appeared. 8 And he sent them to Bethlehem and said, "Go and search carefully for the Child; and when you have found him, report to me, so that I too may come and worship him." 9 After hearing the king, they went their way; and the star, which they had seen in the east, went on before them until it came and stood over the place where the Child was. 10 When they saw the star, they rejoiced exceedingly with great joy. 11 After coming into the house they saw the Child with Mary His mother; and they fell to the ground and worshiped him. Then, opening their treasures, they presented to him gifts of gold,* FRANKINCENSE, *and* **MYRRH.** *12 And having been warned by Yahweh in a dream not to return to Herod, the Magi left for their own country* **by another way***"* [Matthew 2:7-12].

We will emphasize the word **MYRRH** in the fifteen verses throughout the Bible. There will be only three in the *"new testament,"* the first one above. These verses were the first ones quoted in the first section, so I will not repeat the comments of those verses in section two. You may go back and look again in section one; it will refresh your memory.

The **shepherds** came to see Jesus **the very night in which he was born**. However, the magi probably arrived about two years later. He was no longer in a manger – he was in a house, no longer a baby (*paidion*) but a child (*brephos*). They arrived after a very long trip.

That they were the offerings of **three** individuals respectively, each of them **kings**, the very names of whom **tradition** has handed down; - all these are, at the best, **precarious suppositions**. Robertson's Word Pictures says that *"these men may have been Israelite proselytes and may have known of the Messianic hope"* and it probably was.

MYRRH was also a production of Arabia, and was obtained from a tree in the same manner as **FRANKINCENSE**. The name denotes bitterness, and was given to it on account of its great bitterness. It was used chiefly in **embalming the dead**, because it had the property of preserving dead bodies from putrefaction. It was much used in Egypt and in Judea. It was obtained from a thorny tree, which grows 8 or 9 feet high. It was at an early period an article of commerce and was an ingredient of the holy ointment as we have noticed. It was also used as an agreeable perfume. It was also sometimes mingled with wine to form an article of drink. Such a drink was given to the Savior when about to be crucified, as a stupefying potion. The offerings here referred to where it was made because they were the most valuable which the country of the magi or wise men produced. They were tokens of respect and homage which they paid to the king of the Israelites. They proved their high regard for him and their belief that he was to be an illustrious prince. Wise men came from far away to do him homage and bowed down and presented their best gifts and offerings.

Matthew 2:9 indicates that the miraculous star was not always visible to the magi. As they started toward or arrived at Bethlehem, they saw the star **again**; and it led them to the **house** where Jesus was. By now, Joseph had moved Mary and the baby from the temporary dwelling where Jesus had been born (Luke 2:7). The traditional manger scenes that assembled together the shepherds and wise men **are not true to Scripture**. They probably did not find Jesus in Bethlehem and that is the time that the star appeared again and led them to a **house** which was probably in some place in Nazareth, thereby apart from Bethlehem or Jerusalem. Mary lived in Nazareth while she was pregnant with Jesus (Luke 2:4). Oh – do not pass that scripture! Matthew cites a second fulfilled prophecy to prove that Jesus is the king (Matthew 2:5). How he was born was a fulfillment of prophecy. Bethlehem means "*house of bread*," and this was where the "*bread of life*" came to earth. Bethlehem in the "*old* *testament"* was associated with David who was a type of Jesus in his suffering and glory. Here, "*treasures*" means "*caskets*" from the verb *"Titheemi,"* receptacle for valuables. In the ancient writers, it meant "*treasury*" as a "*storehouse.*" Were the wise men always in touch with the star? When did they lose it? Why?

It is likely that the wise men lost sight of it after they had commenced their journey from the East. It is probable that it appeared to them first in the direction of Jerusalem. They concluded that the expected king **had been born**, and immediately commenced their journey to Jerusalem. When they arrived there, it was important that they should be directed to the very place where he was, and the star **again appeared**. It was for this reason that they rejoiced. They felt assured that they were under a heavenly guidance, and would be conducted to the house of the king of the Israelites.

It is supposed that Herod died in the thirty-seventh year of his reign. It is not certainly known in what year he began his reign, and hence it is impossible to determine the time that Joseph remained in Egypt. The best chronologers have supposed that he died somewhere between two and four years after the birth of Jesus, but at what particular time cannot now be determined. Nor can it be ascertained at what age Jesus was taken into Egypt. It seems probable that he was supposed to be a year or two old (see Matthew 2:16), and of course the time that he remained in

Egypt was not long. Herod died of a most painful and loathsome disease in Jericho. This language is recorded in Hosea 11:1. It there evidently speaks of Yahweh's calling His people out of Egypt, under Moses. It might be said to be fulfilled in His calling Jesus from Egypt, because the words in Hosea aptly expressed this also. The same love which led Him to deliver His people Israel from the land of Egypt, now led him also to deliver His Son from that place.

As to the use of **MYRRH**, here is a little information.

This substance is mentioned as valuable for its perfume and as one of the constituents of the holy **incense**.

"Mor" is generally identified with the **MYRRH** of commerce, the dried gum of a species of balsam. This is a stunted tree growing in Arabia, having a light-gray bark; the gum resin exudes in small tear-like drops which dry to a rich brown or reddish-yellow, brittle substance, with a faint though agreeable smell and a warm, bitter taste. It is still used as **medicine** (Mark 15:23). On account, however, of the references to "***flowing MYRRH***" (Exodus 30:23) and "*liquid **MYRRH***" (Song of Solomon 5:5,13), Schweinfurth maintains that *"mor"* was not a dried gum but the liquid balsam of *"Balsamodendron opobalsamum."*

Whichever view is correct, it is probable that the *"smurna,"* of the *"new testament"* was the same. It was brought by the "*wise men*" of the East as an offering to the child Savior. In Mark 15:23 it is offered mingled with wine as an anesthetic to the suffering Redeemer, and in John 19:39 a "*mixture of **MYRRH** and aloes*" is brought by Nicodemus to embalm the body of Jesus.

The **MYRRH** in Genesis 37:25, (*margin "ladanum"* - 43:11), is the fragrant resin obtained from some species of cistus and called in Arabic *"ladham,"* in Latin *"ladanum."* The cistus or "*rock rose*" is exceedingly common all over the mountains of Palestine, the usual varieties having pink petals, and the other with white petals. No commerce is done now in Palestine in this substance as of old, but it is still gathered from various species of cistus, especially C. creticus in the Greek Isles, **where it is collected by threshing the plants** by a kind of flail from which the sticky mass is scraped off with a knife and rolled into **small black balls**. In **Cyprus at the present time** the gum is collected from the **beards of the goats** that browse on these shrubs, as was done in the days of old.

CHAPTER FIFTEEN

<u>MARK 15:23</u>

The second passage in the *"new testament"* is the passage mentioned above which is now quoted …

> <u>*"Then they brought him to the place Golgotha, which is translated, Place of a Skull. 23 They tried to give him wine mixed with* **MYRRH***; but he did not take it"* [NASU].</u>

With that attempt, they crucified Jesus and parted his clothing at 9 AM. On the subject of wine, Matthew says "*vinegar.*" It was probably "*wine soured,*" so that it might be called either. This was the common drink of the Roman soldiers. According to Rabbinic tradition, certain Jerusalem women provided sedative drinks for those about to be crucified, to decrease their pain (cf. Proverbs 31:6-7) …

> <u>*"Give strong drink to him who is perishing, and wine to him whose life is bitter. 7 Let him drink and forget his poverty and remember his trouble no more."*</u>

On arrival at Golgotha, **they**, presumably the Roman soldiers, offered (lit., "*were attempting to give*") Jesus such a drink, wine mixed with **MYRRH**, a plant's sap having **anesthetic properties**. The verb means flavored with **MYRRH**, myrrhed wine. But after he had tasted it (cf. Matthew 27:34) he **refused it**, choosing rather to face suffering and death in full control of all his faculties …

> *"And when they came to a place called Golgotha, which means Place of a Skull, 34 they gave him wine to drink mixed with gall; and **after tasting it**, he was unwilling to drink."*

According to Roman law, the guilty victim had to carry his own cross, or at least the cross beam, to the place of execution, and Jesus was no exception. He left Pilate's hall bearing his cross, but he could not continue; so the soldiers "*drafted*" Simon of Cyrene to carry the cross for him. Roman officers had the privilege of "*impressing*" men for service, and the way they used this privilege irritated the Israelites.

When one considers all that the Lord had endured since his arrest, it is not surprising that his strength failed. Indeed, "*He could have called 10,000 angels,*" yet he willingly bore the suffering on mankind's behalf. There was a higher purpose behind this act; the victim carried the cross because he had been found guilty, but Jesus was not guilty. Mankind was the guilty ones, and Simon carried that cross on their behalf. Simon Peter boasted that he would go with Jesus to prison and to death (Luke 22:33), but it was Simon of Cyrene, not Simon Peter, who came to the aid of their master …

> *"Simon, Simon, behold, satan has demanded permission to sift you like wheat; 32 but I have prayed for you, that your faith may not fail;*

*and you, when once you have turned again, strengthen your brothers." 33 But he said to him, "**Lord, with you I am ready to go both to prison and to death**!" 34 And he said, "I say to you, **Peter**, the rooster will not crow today until you have denied three times that you know me."*

Cyrene was in what is now Libya in North Africa and included a large Israelite community. "*Simon*" was a typical Israelite name and devout Israelite pilgrims from throughout the Mediterranean came to Jerusalem during Passover. Roman soldiers could impress anyone into service to carry things for them. Simon was not coming from "*the field*" (*literally*) as a worker.

The site of the crucifixion <u>**might**</u> have been named "*Place of the Skull*" because so many deaths occurred there. (*The suggestion that the place was shaped like a skull* <u>**is possible**</u>*, but the inference that it is thus the purported site of Calvary proposed by Charles Gordon around 1884 is unlikely; the contours of the ground there were created subsequent to the time of Jesus.*) Many of the ancients mention it as a current tradition, that in this place our first father **<u>Adam was buried</u>**, and they think it highly congruous that there Jesus should be crucified; *"for as in Adam all die, so in Christ shall all be made alive."* But I consider that something more credible is the tradition, that this mount Calvary was that mountain in the land of Moriah (*and in the land of Moriah it certainly was, for so the country about Jerusalem* *was called*), on which Isaac was to be offered; and the ram was offered instead of him; and then Abraham had an eye to this day of Jesus, when he called the place Jehovah-jireh — *"The Lord will provide,"* expecting that so it would be seen in the mount of the Lord.

Pious women of Jerusalem normally prepared a solution like this one and offered it to those being executed to dull their pain (cf. Proverbs 31:6-7); Jesus chose to endure the full force of the agony of crucifixion. **MYRRH** is said to have had narcotic effects.

In addition to the subject of **MYRRH**, it is not strictly **MYRRH** but *"ladanum,"* the resinous exudation of the Cistus (**rock rose**) Creticus, growing in Gilead where no **MYRRH** grew, and exported into Egypt. It is *"odorous, rather green, easy to soften, fat, produced in Cyprus;"* abounding still in Candia (Crete), where they gather it by passing over it an instrument composed of many **parallel leather thongs**, to which its gum adheres.

CHAPTER SIXTEEN

<u>JOHN 19:39</u>

Let us go now to the third and final verse in which **MYRRH** occurs in the *"new testament."* It is as listed in the heading ...

> *"Nicodemus, who had first come to him by night, also came, bringing a mixture of **MYRRH** and aloes, about a hundred pounds weight. 40 So they took the body of Jesus and bound it in linen wrappings with the spices, as is the burial custom of the Israelites."*

Joseph of Arimathea and Nicodemus buried Jesus in the garden where he was crucified; in a new tomb that Joseph had hewn [John 19:39].

MYRRH and aloes are mentioned in this verse. The **drugs** were used to preserve bodies from putrefaction. One scholar says that the **aloes** mentioned here is liquor which runs from an **aromatic** tree, and is **widely different** from that called aloes among us.

The **MYRRH** of Genesis 37:25, was probably *"ladalzum,"* a highly-fragrant resin and volatile oil used as a cosmetic, and stimulative **as a medicine**. It is yielded by the cistus, known in Europe as the rock rose, a shrub with rose-colored flowers, growing in Palestine and along the shores of the Mediterranean.

Some have objected that a hundred pounds' weight of **MYRRH** and aloes was enough to embalm two hundred dead bodies; some critics have proposed to read (*hekateroon*) a mixture of **MYRRH** and aloes, of about a pound **EACH**. But it may be observed that great quantities of spices were used for embalming dead bodies, when they intended to show peculiar marks of respect to the deceased. A great quantity was used at the funeral of Aristobulus; and it is said that five hundred servants bearing aromatics attended the funeral of Herod (see Josephus, Ant. b. 15 c. 3 , s. 4; and b. 17 c. 8 , s. 3); and fourscore pounds of spices were used at the funeral of R. Gamaliel the elder.

Joseph of Arimathea was rich and was waiting for the kingdom. Arimathea was about 20 miles northwest of Jerusalem. Though he was a member of the Sanhedrin, the Israelite council, he was *"a good and upright man who had not consented to their decision"* (Luke 23:50-51). After a crucifixion, the Romans usually left the dead body to the beasts of prey. This lack of proper burial was the final humiliation in a crucifixion. But the Israelites removed exposed bodies. Joseph got permission to bury Jesus' body. He, along with another, influential man, Nicodemus, made the necessary arrangements. About 75 pounds of **MYRRH** and aloes was an extensive amount of spices, used in preparing the body for burial. Perhaps Nicodemus now understood the teaching of Jesus that he would be lifted up and that a man could look in faith to him and live. Both men who had been secret disciples had now became manifest.

Because it was almost the Sabbath (*which began at sundown*) the burial had to take place **quickly**. Israelite burial customs did not involve mummification or embalming, which took out the blood and body organs. Their normal process was to wash the body and cover it with cloth and aromatic oils or spices. The <u>NIV</u> translation of *"othoniois"* as **strips of linen** has some support. However, some Roman Catholic scholars argue for the translation of "*cloth wrappings,*" since Matthew refers to a linen cloth in which Jesus' body was wrapped. Notice the two *"old testament"* passages that were fulfilled in Jesus' death …

> *"Then the Israelites, because it was the day of preparation, so that the bodies would not remain on the cross on the Sabbath (for that Sabbath was a high day), asked Pilate that their legs might be broken, and that they might be taken away. 32 So the soldiers came, and* **broke the legs of the first man** *and of* **the other who was crucified with him**; *33 but coming to Jesus, when they saw that he was already dead, they did not break his legs. 34 But one of the soldiers pierced his side with a spear, and immediately blood and water came out. 35 And he who has seen has testified, and his testimony is true; and he knows that he is telling the truth, so that you also may believe. 36 For these things came to pass to fulfill the Scripture,* **"NOT A BONE OF HIM SHALL BE BROKEN."** *37 And again another Scripture says,* **"THEY SHALL LOOK ON HIM WHOM THEY PIERCED."**

It is remarkable that the Roman soldiers **did not do** what they were commanded to do - break the victims' legs - but **they did do** what they were not supposed to do - pierce the Savior's side! In both matters, they fulfilled the very words of Yahweh! The bones of the Passover lamb were not to be broken (Exodus 12:46; Numbers 9:12; and note Psalms 34:20), so the Lord's bones were protected by Yahweh. His side was to be pierced (Zechariah 12:10; Revelation 1:7), so that was done by one of the soldiers. Had the two believers who buried Jesus not been there, Jesus would have been carried to the valley of Hinnom or Gehenna and let the perpetual fire destroy it. Of course, when the two men touched Jesus' dead body, they defiled themselves and could not participate in Passover. Mary of Bethany had already anointed Jesus' body for burial (Mark 14:8; John 12:1-8).

The writer saw a special significance to the blood and water that came from the wound in Jesus' side. For one thing, it proved that Jesus had a real body and experienced a real death. By the time the writer wrote this book, there were false teachers in the assembly claiming that Jesus did not have a truly human body. There may also be a **symbolic meaning** - the blood speaks of justification, the water of sanctification and cleansing. The blood takes care of the **guilt** of sin; the water deals with the **stain** of sin. As far as we know, of all the disciples, **only (~~John~~) Lazarus** was with them at the cross. Jesus had finished the work of the "*new creation*" (2 Corinthians 5:17), and now he would rest.

CHAPTER SEVENTEEN

GENESIS 37:25

Well, we have covered the three verses in the *"new testament,"* so we will go back to the twelve verses of the *"old testament."* We will begin with the one of the heading of this chapter. Here it is ...

> *"Then they sat down to eat a meal. And as they raised their eyes and looked, behold, a caravan of Ishmaelites was coming from Gilead, with their camels bearing* **aromatic gum** *(***FRANKINCENSE***?) and balm (***aloes***?) and* **MYRRH**, *on their way to bring them down to Egypt. 26* **Judah** *said to his brothers, "What profit is it for us to kill our brother and cover up his blood? 27 "Come and let us sell him to the Ishmaelites and not lay our hands on him, for he is our brother, our own flesh." And his brothers listened to him. 28 Then some* **Midianite** *traders passed by, so they pulled him up and lifted Joseph out of the pit, and sold him to the Ishmaelites for* **twenty shekels of silver**. *Thus they brought Joseph into Egypt."*

"*A caravan of Ishmaelite Arabs came.*" This seems to give the true sense. Since there were only eight (*Reubin was absent at the sale*) of the brethren present, and they sold Joseph for twenty shekels (*8 ounces of silver*), each had more than two shekels as his share in this most infamous transaction. The merchants paid **twenty** pieces of silver; and the price of a slave in Egypt being **thirty** pieces of silver – says <u>Josephus</u>. **MYRRH** was part of the cargo of the caravan.

Trading in the produce of Arabia and India, they were, in the regular course of traffic, on their way to Egypt; and the chief articles of commerce in which trading caravans dealt were a strong fragrant perfume called storax, and hence, applied generally to spicery and **all kinds of aromatic substances**, from India and Ceylon - sweet odors, **incense** and balm, distilled from a shrub in Gilead, **famous for its medicinal properties**, and frequently mentioned in Scripture; and **MYRRH**, the resinous gum of a small odoriferous tree, Cistus creticus, growing in Arabia-Felix and North Africa, celebrated as a **perfume and stimulating medicine**, and often given as a present, on account of its value and rarity. For these articles there must have been an enormous demand in Egypt, as they were constantly used in the process of embalmment.

It must have given the brothers great pleasure to strip Joseph of his special robe **of many colors** and then drop him into the empty cistern. Cisterns were usually quite deep and had long narrow openings that would be too high for a prisoner to reach. In order to get out, you would need somebody to lower a rope and pull you up.

It is difficult to understand how the brothers could sit down and calmly eat a meal while their brother was suffering and begging them to set him free. However, hearts that have been hardened by hatred and poisoned by thoughts of murder are not likely to pay much attention to the cries of their victim. But then, think of what the Lord's own nation did to him! All of us are potentially capable of doing what Joseph's brothers did, for *"the heart is deceitful above all things, and desperately wicked: who can know it"* (Jeremiah 17:9 - <u>KJV</u>)?

Just then, the brothers spied a Midianite merchant train moving across the plain, and this gave them an idea. They could sell their brother as a **slave** and at the same time get rid of him and make some money. Sound familiar? Since anybody taken to Egypt and sold for a slave was not likely to win his freedom and come back again, there was no danger that their plot would ever be discovered. They forgot that Yahweh was watching and was still in control. Jacob had inherited the covenant blessings and this made him a very special person in the eyes of Yahweh. The Lord had His divine purposes to fulfill, and *"there is no wisdom or understanding or counsel against the Lord"* (Proverbs 21:30 - <u>NKJV</u>).

Starting with Cain's murder of Abel, *"man's inhumanity to man"* is painfully recorded in both biblical and secular history. We are made in the image of Yahweh, and we belong to the same human family, and yet **<u>we can not seem to get along with one another</u>**. Everything from family feuds over lottery winnings to civil wars blamed on ancient injuries gives evidence that the **world desperately needs a Savior who can make hearts new**.

Reuben was absent when his brothers sold Joseph, perhaps taking care of some **problem with the sheep**. When he visited the cistern, he was shocked to find that Joseph was gone. Thus he hurried back to the camp to find out what had happened. Certainly his attitude and actions made it clear to his brothers that **his sympathies were with Joseph, for he tore his clothes like a man in mourning**.

By the law of the *"go'el,"* the **oldest was constituted protector** of his younger brother; hence, finding that Joseph was not in the pit, he rent his clothes, and uttered that wail which, in Hebrew, is so touching from its sounds: **"The child is not, and I, whither shall I go."** His excessive grief arose from a sense of his personal responsibility. His intentions were excellent, and his feelings no doubt were painful when he discovered what had been done in his absence. But the thing was of Yahweh.

"He who covers his sins will not prosper" (Proverbs 28:13 - <u>NKJV</u>) is Yahweh's unchanging law, but people still think they can defy it and escape the consequences. Among Jacob's sons, one sin led to another as the brothers fabricated the evidence that would deceive their father into thinking that Joseph was dead, killed by a wild beast. Jacob would have no problem identifying the **special robe**, and he would have no way to test the blood. As

tragic and treacherous as this deception was, **Jacob was reaping what he himself had sown**.

Years before, he had killed a goat in order to deceive his father (Genesis 27:1-17); and now his own sons were following in his footsteps. Unwilling to confront their father **personally**, the brothers **sent a servant** to Jacob to show him the "*evidence*" and tell him the lie that they had concocted. This was a **brutal** way to treat their father, but "*the tender mercies of the wicked are cruel*" (Proverbs 12:10 - NKJV). Prone to jump to conclusions (Genesis 32:6-8), Jacob accepted the evidence, believed the story, and concluded that Joseph indeed was dead. He went into deep mourning, and **twenty years later was still grieving over the death** of Joseph (42:36). His family tried to comfort him, but to no avail. His favorite son was dead, and Jacob would carry his grief with him to the grave.

Years later, Jacob would lament, "*All these things are against me*" (v-36 - KJV), when actually all those things were working for him. This does not mean that Yahweh approved of or engineered the brothers' hatred and deception, or that they were not responsible for what they did. It does mean that Yahweh is so great that He can work out His purposes even when people are doing their worst. The greatest example of this is Calvary. Years later, Joseph would say, "*You meant evil against me; but Yahweh meant it for good*" (Genesis 50:20 - NKJV).

Yahweh providentially brought Joseph safely to Egypt and saw to it that he was sold to one of Pharaoh's chief officers. **Potiphar** is called "*captain of the guard,*" which suggests that he was head of Pharaoh's personal bodyguard and in charge of official executions. But the important thing was not that Joseph was connected with such a powerful man in Egypt. The important thing was that "*the Lord was with Joseph and he prospered*" (39:2). What a view does this exhibit of those hardened brothers! Their **common share** in this conspiracy is not the only dismal feature in the story. The almost instantaneous manner in which the proposal was followed by their joint resolution, and the cool indifference, or rather the fiendish satisfaction, with which they **sat down to feed themselves**, is astonishing; it is impossible that mere envy at his dreams, his gaudy dress, or the partiality of their common father, could have goaded them on to such a pitch of frenzied resentment, or confirmed them in such wickedness. Their **hatred to Joseph** must **have had a far deeper seat** - must have been produced by dislike to his piety and other excellences, which made his character and conduct a constant censure upon theirs, and on account of which they found that they could never be at ease until they had rid themselves of his hated presence. This was the true solution of the mystery, just as it was in the case of Cain (1 John 3:12).

CHAPTER EIGHTEEN

GENESIS 43:11

This chapter is a follow-up with the sons of Jacob having been accused of Joseph, as second in command under Pharaoh, of stealing. But the Israelites had nowhere to go for food, so they complied with Joseph which they had not recognized. Here is the passage listed above ...

> *"Then their father Israel said to them, "If it must be so, then do this: take some of the best products of the land in your bags, and carry down to the man as a present, a little balm and a little honey, **aromatic gum and MYRRH**, pistachio nuts and almonds. 12 "Take double the money in your hand, and take back in your hand the money that was returned in the mouth of your sacks; perhaps it was a mistake. 13 "Take your brother also, and arise, return to the man; 14 and may Yahweh Almighty grant you compassion in the sight of the man, so that he will release to you your other brother and Benjamin. And as for me, if I am bereaved of my children, I am bereaved." 15 So the men took this present, and they took double the **money** in their hand, **and Benjamin**; then they arose and went down to Egypt and stood before Joseph."*

The children if Israel were to carry down a present to Joseph. From the very earliest times, presents were used as means of introduction to great men. This is particularly noticed by Solomon: *"A man's gift maketh room for him, and bringeth him before great men*" (Proverbs 18:16). But what was the present that was brought to Joseph on this occasion? After all the labor of commentators, we are obliged to be contented with probabilities and conjectures. According to our translation, the gifts were balm, honey, spices, **MYRRH**, nuts, and almonds.

Balm is supposed to signify resin in general, or some kind of gum issuing from trees. Honey has been supposed to be the same as **the rob of grapes**, called in Egypt **dibs**. Others think that honey, in the common sense of the term, is to be understood here; we know that honey was plentiful in Palestine. Spices are supposed to mean gum storax which might be very valuable on account of its qualities as a perfume. **MYRRH** is supposed by some to mean stacte, by others to signify an ointment made of **MYRRH**. Nuts, by some rendered pistachio nuts, those produced in Syria being the finest in the world; by others, dates; others, walnuts, others, pine apples, others, the nuts of the terebinth tree. Almonds, correctly enough translated, and perhaps the only article in the collection of which we know anything with certainty. It is generally allowed that the land of Canaan produces the best almonds in the east; and on this account they might be deemed a very acceptable present to the governor of Egypt.

The Israelites were to double money. What was returned in their sacks and what was further **necessary to buy another load of food**.

Benjamin went down to Egypt with his brothers. Interestingly, Judah was the one who had come up with the plan to sell Joseph to Egypt. Now he had to negotiate with his father in order to get Benjamin to see Joseph. Jacob suggested that they take some of their best products to the man as a gift. Apparently, those delicacies were not available in Egypt. They also took double the amount of silver, returning what they had found in their money pouches before. Jacob resigned himself to the high risk involved in possibly losing a third son - first, Joseph; then Simeon; and now perhaps Benjamin too.

The restored money in the sack's mouth was a perplexing circumstance. But it might have been done **inadvertently by one of the servants** - so Jacob persuaded himself; and happy it was for his own peace and the encouragement of the travelers that he took this view. Besides the duty of restoring it, **honesty** in their case was clearly the best, **the safest policy**.

As we noted, the famine continued and Jacob's family needed more grain. This time, however, Benjamin had to go with them to Egypt. Judah reminded his father that without Benjamin their long trip to Egypt would be in vain. Jacob was, of course, reluctant; his scolding (*why did you tell the man you had another brother?*) was an effort to escape the decision he dreaded to make. Yet he must release Benjamin so they could return to Egypt. Otherwise they would **all die from starvation**. Jacob probably asked the sons **why did you tell Joseph that you had another brother**?

It is not a fault, but our wisdom and duty is to alter our purposes and resolutions when there is a good reason for our so doing as was Jacob's. **Constancy is a virtue, but obstinacy is not**. It is Yahweh's prerogative not to repent, and to make unchangeable resolves (Genesis 43:11-14).

The famine was sore in Canaan and yet they had balm and **MYRRH**, etc.. We may live well enough upon plain food without dainties; but we cannot live upon dainties without plain food. Let us thank Yahweh that which is most needful and useful is generally cheap and common. Sometimes we must not think it too much to **buy peace** even where **we may justly demand it**, and insist upon it as our right.

CHAPTER NINETEEN

EXODUS 30:23

With the next verse that contains the word **MYRRH**, it is in conjunction with the Israelite sanctuary. Here is the paragraph listed above ...

*"Moreover, the Lord spoke to Moses, saying, 23 "Take also for yourself the finest of spices: of **flowing MYRRH** five hundred shekels, and of fragrant cinnamon half as much, two hundred and fifty, and of fragrant cane two hundred and fifty, 24 and of cassia five hundred, according to the shekel of the sanctuary, and of olive oil a hin. 25 "You shall make of these a holy anointing oil, a perfume mixture, the work of a perfumer; it shall be a holy anointing oil. 26 "With it you shall anoint the tent of meeting and the ark of the testimony, 27 and the table and all its utensils, and the lampstand and its utensils, and the altar of incense, 28 and the altar of burnt offering and all its utensils, and the laver and its stand. 29 "You shall also consecrate them, that they may be most holy; **whatever touches them shall be holy.** 30 "You shall **anoint Aaron and his sons,** and consecrate them, that they may minister as priests to Me. 31 "You shall speak to the sons of Israel, saying, **'This shall be a holy anointing oil to Me** throughout your generations. 32 'It shall not be poured on anyone's body, nor shall you make any like it in the same proportions; it is holy, and it shall be holy to you. 33 'Whoever shall mix any like it or whoever puts any of it on a layman shall be **cut off from his people."***

Yahweh had said to take also unto them principal spices. From this and the following verse we learn that **the holy anointing oil was compounded** of the following ingredients.

The original *"roqach,"* signifies *"a compounder or confectioner; any person who compounds drugs, aromatics,"* etc.. The compound was pure **MYRRH**; 500 shekels - *MYRRH* is the product of an oriental tree **not well known**, and is collected by making an incision in the tree. What is now called by this name **is precisely the same as that of the ancients**. Pure means *"free flowing;"* also sweet cinnamon and sweet calamus (or cane).

It was Yahweh's desire that the nation of Israel be *"a kingdom of priests"* in the world, revealing His glory and sharing His blessings with the unbelieving nations around them. But in order to magnify a holy Yahweh, **Israel had to be a holy people**, and that is where the Aaronic priesthood came in. It was the task of the priests (*Aaron's family*) and the Levites to serve in the tabernacle and represent the people before Yahweh. The priests were also to represent Yahweh to the people by teaching them the law and helping them to obey it.

But Israel failed to live like a kingdom of priests. Instead, the spiritual leadership in the nation gradually deteriorated until the priests actually permitted the people to worship idols in the temple of Yahweh (Ezekiel 8)! The Lord punished His people by allowing the Babylonians to destroy Jerusalem and the temple and carry thousands of Israelites into exile. Why did this happen? *"But it happened because of the sins of her prophets and the iniquities of her priests, who shed within her the blood of the righteous"* (Lamentations 4:13 - <u>NIV</u>).

It was stated that Moses was to take of olive oil a hin. Strange word here. <u>**Hin**</u> is a word of Egyptian origin, equal to ten pints. It was originally the general name for a vessel, which was then transferred by the Hebrews and Egyptians to a certain measure of variable compass. Being mixed with the olive oil - no doubt of the purest kind - this composition probably remained always in a liquid state; and in order to separate what was sacred from common application either for food or luxury, the strictest prohibition issued against using it for any other purpose than anointing the tabernacle and its furniture. **<u>There is no record of the temple being anointed as the tabernacle was</u>**. According to Israelite tradition, there was no holy oil in the second temple; and the formal ceremony of anointing was probably omitted at the dedication of the first (*Solomon's*) temple in consequence of the removal from the tabernacle to that permanent building, of the sacred vessels which had been previously anointed.

Directions are here given for the composition of the holy anointing oil and the incense (***<u>FRANKINCENSE and MYRRH</u>***) that were to be used in the service of the tabernacle; with these Yahweh was to be honored, and therefore He would appoint the making of them; for nothing comes to Yahweh but what comes from Him. The holy anointing oil is here ordered to be made up with the ingredients and their quantities as prescribed (vs-23-25). Interpreters are not agreed concerning them but we are sure, in general, that they were the best and fittest for the purpose; they must need be so when the divine wisdom appointed them for the divine honor. It was to be compounded *"after the art of the apothecary"* (v-25). The spices were in all nearly half a hundred weight, were to be infused in the oil, which was to be about five or six quarts, and then strained out, leaving an admirable sweet smell in the oil. With this oil, Yahweh's tent and all the furniture were to be anointed. It was to be used also in the consecration of the priests (v- 26-30). It was to be continued throughout their generations (v-31).

CHAPTER TWENTY

ESTHER 2:12

Esther, who was part of the king's harem, was made the **king's wife** instead of Vashti. The following is the verse that contains **MYRRH** in the next verse of our study ...

*"Now when the turn of each young lady came to go in to King Ahasuerus, after the end of her twelve months under the regulations for the women — for the days of their beautification were completed as follows: six months with oil of **MYRRH** and six months with spices and the cosmetics for women — 13 the young lady would go in to the king in this way; anything that she desired was given her to take with her from the harem to the king's palace. 14 In the evening she would go in and in the morning she would return to the **second harem**, to the custody of Shaashgaz, the king's eunuch who was in charge of the concubines. She would not again go in to the king unless the king delighted in her **and she was summoned by name**. 15 Now when the turn of Esther, the daughter of Abihail the uncle of Mordecai who had taken her as his daughter, came to go in to the king, she did not request anything except what Hegai, the king's eunuch who was in charge of the women, advised. And **Esther found favor in the eyes of all who saw her**. 16 So Esther was taken to King Ahasuerus to his royal palace in the tenth month which is the month Tebeth, in the seventh year of his reign."*

Esther was six months with the oil of **MYRRH**. See Esther 2:3 and we will quote that verse ...

> *"And let the king appoint officers in all the provinces of his kingdom, that they may gather together all the fair young virgins unto Shushan the palace, to **the house of the women**, unto the custody of Hege the king's chamberlain, keeper of the women; and let their things for **purification** be given them."*

Hege was the king's chamberlain or "*Hege, the king's **eunuch**;*" so the Septuagint, the Vulgate, the Targum and the Syriac. In the Eastern countries the women are entrusted to the care of the **eunuchs only**.

The things for purification were given to them and their cosmetics. What these were, we are told in the verse that we quoted; oil of **MYRRH** and sweet odors. The **MYRRH** was employed for six months, and the odors for six months more; after which the person was brought to the king. This **space was sufficient to show** whether the young woman had been chaste; whether she was with child or not, that the king might not be imposed on, and be obliged to father an illegitimate offspring, which might have been the case had not this precaution been used.

Some say that instead of the oil of **MYRRH**, the Targum says it was the oil of **unripe olives**, which **caused the hair to fall off, and rendered the skin delicate**. Esther's skin being delicate would be good but baldness of her head would not be good — therefore I have a hard time with this supposition. The reason of this purification seems **not** to be apprehended by any writer I have seen.

Esther was one of the children of the captivity, an Israelite woman and a sharer with her people in their bondage. The most beautiful of all the **young virgins** of all the provinces of Babylon were to be selected, and those were taken out of all classes of the people, indiscriminately, consequently there must have been many who were brought up in low life. Now we know that those who feed on coarse and strong food, which is **not easily digested**, have generally an abundant perspiration (*sweat*), which is **strongly odorous**, and in many, though in every respect amiable, and even beautiful, this odor is **far from being pleasant**. Pure, wholesome, easily digested and nourishing aliment, with the frequent use of the hot bath, continued for twelve months, **the body frequently rubbed with olive oil**, will in almost every case remove all that is disagreeable of this kind. This treatment will give a healthy action to all the internal vessels, and in every respect promote health and comfort.

She required nothing when she went into the king. The other virgins perhaps loaded themselves with precious ornaments of various kinds, necklaces, bracelets, earrings, anklets and the like. Esther let Hegai dress her as he would. When she went into the king, he loved her above all so he set the royal crown upon her head and made her what is now called in the East the **SULTANA**,

the queen. She was the mistress of all the rest of the wives, all of whom were obliged to pay her the most profound respect. (Esther 2:12-15; Esther 2:16-20; Esther 2:21-23.) Esther became extremely popular during her year of preparation for her night with the king. Each girl's beauty treatments were designed to enhance her attractiveness. **Myrrh**, a gum from a small tree, gives a fragrant smell.

Esther was not in a beauty contest simply to win the king's affections; the women were being prepared to have sexual relations with the king. This is suggested by the words in the evening she would go there and in the morning return. After that, they would be transferred to another harem, under Shaash-gaz, which consisted of the concubines. Most of the women were relegated to living the rest of their lives in the harem of the concubines, many probably never again seeing the king. When Esther went to the king, she followed the instructions of Hegai the eunuch.

Esther was taken to the King in 479 B.C., his seventh year - the 10th month. The king was attracted to Esther and therefore made her queen in place of Vashti. Then a big banquet was prepared and he proclaimed a holiday and gave away many gifts. Throughout all this, **Esther had still not revealed that she belonged to the Israelite nation** (cf. v-10). Apparently, there was a gathering of **another harem of virgins** during the time

Mordecai was at the king's gate. His being at the king's gate, probably meant that Mordecai held an official position in the empire's judicial system. His position thus helped set the stage for the following events. This fact about Mordecai shows how he could have **uncovered an assassination plot and how a feud started that threatened the entire Israelite nation**. Many have noted that the <u>Book of Esther</u> is a great short story. Like Ruth, another little book in the Bible about a woman, Esther has all the earmarks of great literature, including a conflict, an antagonist, tension and irony. The antagonist, Haman, is introduced here and his conflict with Mordecai began. Again a reference to Mordecai's position at the king's gate as a judiciary official points to **Yahweh's sovereign control over these events**. Learning about a plot by Bigthana and Teresh, royal guards, to assassinate the king, Mordecai told Queen Esther, who reported this to the king. She gave credit to Mordecai for uncovering the scheme. The two men involved in the plot were hanged on a gallows (*or* "***post***," <u>NIV</u> marg.; cf. 5:14). Rather than being hanged by the neck on a modern-type gallows, the men were **probably impaled** on a stake or post. This was **not an unusual method of execution in the Persian Empire.** Darius, Xerxes' father, was known to have once impaled 3,000 men. A record of this assassination attempt was written in the annals, the official royal record (cf. Esther 6:1-2).

Each night, a new maiden was brought to the king; and in the morning, she was sent to the **house of the concubines**, never again to be with the king unless he remembered her and called for her. Such unbridled sensuality eventually would have so bored the king that he was probably unable to distinguish one maiden from another. This was not love. It was faceless, anonymous lust that craved more and more; and the more the king indulged, the less he was satisfied.

Esther had won the favor of everybody who saw her; and when the king saw her, he responded to her with greater enthusiasm than he had to any of the other women. **At last he had found someone to replace Vashti**! The phrase "*the king loved Esther*" (<u>KJV</u>) must not be interpreted to mean that the king had suddenly fallen in love with Esther with pure and devoted affection. The <u>NIV</u> rendering is best: "*Now the king was attracted to Esther more than to any of the other women*" (v-17). **This response was from the Lord who wanted Esther in the royal palace where she could intercede for her people**. "*Known to Yahweh from eternity are all His works*" (Acts 15:18 - <u>NKJV</u>).

It is worth noting that Esther put herself into the hands of Hegai and did what she was told to do. Hegai knew what the king liked, and, being partial to Esther, he attired her accordingly. Because she possessed such great beauty "*in form and features*" (Esther

2:7 - <u>NIV</u>), Esther did not require the "*extras*" that the other women needed.

The king personally crowned Esther and named her the new queen of the empire not knowing that she was one of the children of the captivity, **an Israelite woman** and a sharer with her people in their bondage. She was an orphan; her father and mother were both dead (v-7), but, when they had forsaken her, then the Lord took her up. Her wisdom and virtue were her greatest beauty, but it is an advantage to be a diamond. Mordecai, her cousin-german, was her guardian, brought her up, and took her for his own daughter. The LXX says that he designed to make her his wife. Then he summoned his officials and hosted a great banquet. (*This is the fourth banquet in the book. The Persian kings used every opportunity to celebrate!*) But the king's generosity even touched the common people, for he proclaimed a national holiday throughout his realm and distributed gifts to the people. This holiday may have been similar to the Hebrew "*Year of Jubilee.*" It is likely that **taxes were canceled, servants set free, and workers given a vacation** from their jobs. The king wanted everybody to feel good about his new queen.

The second "*gathering of the virgins*" mentioned in verse 19 probably means that the king's officers continued to gather beautiful girls for his harem, for the king was not likely to become a monogamist and spend the rest of his life with Esther **alone**. Those who hold that this entire occasion was a "*beauty contest*," see this second gathering as a farewell to the "*candidates*" who never got to see the king. **They were thanked and sent home**. I prefer the first interpretation. Queen or no queen, **a man like the king was not about to release a group of beautiful virgins from his palace**!

But most importantly, in verse 19, we now see Mordecai in a position of honor and authority, sitting at the king's gate. In the East, **the gate** was the ancient equivalent of our modern **law courts**, the place where important official business was transacted. It is possible that Queen Esther **used her influence to get her cousin** this job.

Once again, we marvel at the providence of Yahweh in the life of a man who was not honoring the Yahweh of Israel. **Neither Mordecai nor Esther had revealed their true nationality** – Israelites. Perhaps we should classify them with Nicodemus and Joseph of Arimathea who were "*secret disciples*" and yet were used by Yahweh to protect and bury the body of Jesus. Like these two people, Mordecai and Esther were "*hidden*" in the Persian capital because Yahweh had a very special work for them to do. Mordecai was able to use his position for the good of both the king and the Israelites. In Eastern courts, palace intrigue was a normal thing. Only a few officers had free access to the king (*like the White House*), and they often used their privileges to get **bribes** from people who needed the king's help (*like our government*). This is why Daniel's fellow officers did not like him; **he was too honest**.

It is possible that this assassination attempt was connected with the crowning of the new queen and that Vashti's supporters in the palace resented what the king had done. Or perhaps those two men hated Esther because she was an outsider. Although it was not consistently obeyed, tradition said that Persian kings should select their wives from women within the seven noble families of the land. These conspirators may have been traditionalists who did not want a "*commoner*" on the throne.

The king enjoyed almost unlimited authority, wealth and pleasure (*like our president*). He was insulated from the everyday problems of life; but this did not guarantee his personal safety. It was still possible for people to plot against the king and threaten his life. In fact, fourteen years later, the king was assassinated!

Yahweh, in His providence, enabled Mordecai to hear about the plot and notify Queen Esther. When Esther told the king, she gave Mordecai the credit for uncovering the conspiracy; and this meant that his name was written into the official chronicle. This fact will play an important part in the drama four years later (6:1 ff).

The phrase "*hanged on a tree*" probably means "*impaled on a stake*," one of the usual forms of capital punishment used by the Persians, who were not known for their leniency to prisoners. The usual form of capital punishment among the Israelites was stoning; but if they really wanted to humiliate the victim, they would hang the corpse on a tree until sundown.

Mordecai received neither recognition nor reward for saving the king's life. No matter; Yahweh saw to it that the facts were permanently recorded, and He would make good use of them at the right time. Our good works are like seeds that are **planted by faith** and their fruits do not always appear immediately. "*Evil pursues sinners, but to the righteous, good shall be repaid*" (Proverbs 13:21 - <u>NKJV</u>). Joseph befriended a fellow prisoner, and the man completely forgot his kindness for two years (Genesis 40:23; 41:1). **But Yahweh's timing is always perfect, and He sees to it that no good deed is ever wasted**. The plot that Mordecai successfully exposed, however, was nothing compared to the plot he would uncover four years later, planned and perpetrated by Haman, **the enemy of the Israelites**.

As far as Esther is concerned, a whole year was spent in preparation for the intended honor. Considering that this **took place in a palace**, the long period prescribed, **together with the profusion of costly and fragrant cosmetics** employed, was probably required by state etiquette. At the same time, it is said that from the dirty and neglected way in which the girls were brought up in their humble homes, a long process of purification was absolutely necessary before those celebrated beauties were fit for being brought into the markets. Reasons of a similar kind may have originated the cleansing processes. But fragrant perfumes were an indispensable mark of royal gratification to the kings of Persia. In fact, perfumes were used profusely, **without regard either to cost or to quality**.

CHAPTER TWENTY-ONE

SONG OF SOLOMON 1:13

The remainder of the verses in the Bible that uses the word **MYRRH** are found in the book that we call <u>Song of Solomon</u> – which there are **eight**. We will look at them in succession. The first one is the heading of this chapter. I quote …

> *"If you yourself do not know, most beautiful among women, go forth on the trail of the flock and pasture your young goats by the tents of the shepherds. 9 "To me, my darling, you are like my mare among the chariots of Pharaoh. 10 "Your cheeks are lovely with ornaments, your neck with strings of beads." 11 "We will make for you ornaments of gold with beads of silver." 12 "While the king was at his table, my perfume gave forth its fragrance. 13 "My beloved is to me a pouch of **MYRRH** which lies all night between my breasts. 14 "My beloved is to me a cluster of henna blossoms in the vineyards of Engedi." 15 "How beautiful you are, my darling, how beautiful you are! Your eyes are like doves." 16 "How handsome you are, my beloved, and so pleasant! Indeed, our couch is luxuriant! 17 "The beams of our houses are cedars, our rafters, cypresses."*

This and the next Song-sections are regarded by ancient commentators (*Israelites and Christians*) as expressing "*the love of espousals*" between the Holy One and His assembly, first in the wilderness of the Exodus and then in the wilderness of the world.

In verse 9, it reads as this translation records. This should be translated, more literally, "*I have compared thee to my **mare** (not horses) in the chariots or courses of Pharaoh;*" and so the versions understood it. As applied to the bride, it expresses the stately and imposing character of her beauty.

A dialogue ensues between the king and the bride, in which each in succession develops the thought or returns the commendations of the other. Almost every term of praise and endearment here employed may be exactly paralleled by those elsewhere made use of in Scripture to describe the relations of Israel to the heavenly Bridegroom. Public communion with him at the table amidst his friends is spoken of; **primarily in the Israelite assembly**. The allegory supposes the king to have stopped in his movements and to be seated with his friends on the couch.

Outward beauty is of course the first here thought of; but this outward fairness is **the symbol and accompaniment** of an inward beauty indicated in the words "*thine eyes are doves,*" i.e., innocent, meek and loving. The bride is herself called "*a dove*" throughout this book as is the assembly of Israel.

Though she recognized his physical good looks (*handsome*) she was more taken by the charm of his personality (*Oh, how charming!*). The word "*charming*" means "*pleasant*" or "*lovely*" and the combination, handsome and pleasant, was as rare then as it is now. This is the first of about two dozen times she referred to him as **my lover**. The beams of cedars and the rafters made of firs probably **do not refer** to a literal building **but figuratively** to the setting in which they first met. This is also suggested by the verdant (*green*) bed (*couch*). The field where they fell in love and sat talking **was green** and she was given in marriage in the Hebrew dialect.

The lover returned her praise by commending not only her beauty (*beautiful occurs twice in this verse*) but also her tranquil character. In antiquity, doves were noted for their cleanliness and tranquility. "*According to Rabbinic teaching, a bride who has beautiful eyes possesses a beautiful character; they are an index to her character.*"

It is the bundle of **MYRRH** which the bride says shall lie all night between her breasts, to which she compares the bridegroom, his name being as pleasing and refreshing to her mind, as the **MYRRH** or stacte was to her senses, **by its continual fragrance**.

A bundle of **MYRRH** - implied abundant preciousness. So the Greek for "*precious*" is literally, preciousness. Even a little **MYRRH** was very costly, much more a bundle. Sanctius takes it of a scent-box filled with liquid **MYRRH**; the liquid obtained by incision gave the tree its chief value.

Most interpreters, **ignoring the lessons of botany**, explain v-13 of a **little bunch** of **MYRRH**; but whence could the bride obtain this **MYRRH**?

In Palestine, that which is aromatic in the **MYRRH are the leaves and flowers**, but the resin cannot be tied in a bunch. Thus the **MYRRH** here can be understood in no other way than as in general, properly denoting not what one binds up together, but what one ties up - thus a little bag. It is not supposed that she carried such a little bag with her or a box of **FRANKINCENSE**; but she **compares her beloved** to a **MYRRH**-repository, which day and night departs not from her bosom, and penetrates her inwardly with its heart-strengthening aroma. So constantly does she think of him, and so delightful is it for her to dare to think of him **as her beloved**.

She says that her beloved is to her **internally** what such a cluster of cypress-flowers would be to her **externally**. To be able to call him **her beloved** is her ornament; and to **think of him refreshes her like the most fragrant flowers**.

The expression *"Our bed is green"* is the epithet that is appropriate for a bank or natural bed of grass and flowers - like a mattress.

The "*night*" was the whole present dispensation until the everlasting day dawned in 74 A.D.. Thus, this entire story is probably about Jesus and his bride – his beloved!

CHAPTER TWENTY-TWO

SONG OF SOLOMON 3:6

Read the passage below and you will find that it is almost the same as in one of the other chapters. The reading is the passage of this chapter's heading. I quote …

> *"What is this coming up from the wilderness like columns of smoke, perfumed with **MYRRH** and **FRANKINCENSE**, with all scented powders of the merchant? 7 "Behold, it is the traveling couch of Solomon; sixty mighty men around it, of the mighty men of Israel. 8 "All of them are wielders of the sword, expert in war; each man has his sword at his side, guarding against the terrors of the night. 9 "King Solomon has made for himself a sedan chair from the timber of Lebanon. 10 "He made its posts of silver, its back of gold and its seat of purple fabric, with its interior lovingly fitted out by the daughters of Jerusalem. 11 "Go forth, O daughters of Zion, and gaze on King Solomon with the crown with which his mother has crowned him on the day of his wedding, and on the day of his gladness of heart."*

As the other passage that we quoted, this paragraph is about Solomon's wedding day. Going to Egypt was called descending or **going down**, coming from it was termed **coming up**. The bride, having risen, goes after her spouse to the country, and the clouds of **INCENSE** (**_MYRRH_** and **_FRANKINCENSE_**) arising from her court seemed like pillars of smoke; and the appearance was altogether so splendid as to attract the admiration of her own women, who converse about her splendor, excellence, etc., and then take occasion to describe Solomon's nuptial bed and chariot. Some think that it is the bridegroom who is spoken of here.

The sixty men were the guards about the pavilion of the bridegroom, who were placed there because of fear in the night. The security and state of the prince required such a guard as that, and the passage is to be literally understood. As we have studied, they are swordsmen. Every man has a sword and is well instructed how to use it.

The part that is paved with love was a superb piece of embroidery, wrought by some of the noble maids of Jerusalem, and, as a proof of their affection, respect and love, presented to the bride and bridegroom on their nuptial day. This is most likely to be the sense of the passage, though some suppose it to refer to the **whole court**. And as this was done by the **daughters of Jerusalem**, they might have expressed the most striking parts of such a chaste history of love. This chariot was of Solomon's own contriving and making, the materials very rich, **silver, gold, cedar and purple**. He made it for himself, and yet made it for the daughters of Jerusalem, to oblige them. The call that was given to the daughters of Zion to acquaint themselves with the glories of King Solomon, says to go forth and behold him. The multitude of the spectators adds to the beauty of a splendid cavalcade.

This is the exhortation of the companions of the bride to the females of the city to examine the superb appearance of the bridegroom, and especially the nuptial crown, which appears to have been made by Bathsheba, who it is supposed might have lived until the time of Solomon's marriage with the daughter of Pharaoh. It is conjectured that the prophet refers to a nuptial crown. But a crown, both on the bride and bridegroom, was common among most people on such occasions. However, the nuptial crown among the Greeks and Romans was only a wreath of flowers. The elaborate wedding procession, which at first appeared in the distance to be great **pillars of smoke**, is an image of delight and pleasure. **FRANKINCENSE**, **MYRRH** and other perfumes are burned in such abundance around the bridal group that the whole procession appears from the distance to be one of moving wreaths and columns of smoke. "*Who is this*?" The Hebrew is **feminine**, and must refer to the bride riding in the Bridegroom's chariot.

The bride (*wife*) and the king are enjoying a "*mountaintop experience*" as they share their love and he tells her how beautiful she is. It could be translated "*love-making*." He rejoices that his bride is a virgin, "*a garden locked up, a spring enclosed and a fountain sealed.*" This is another evidence that the Lord wants both the man and the woman to stay sexually pure. Conjugal love is pictured in terms of satisfying thirst and exploring a beautiful and fruitful garden that never grows old. The bride is the garden, and the bridegroom prays that the winds of life will make her even more beautiful and desirable.

The *"new testament"* says that one greater than Solomon was there in Jesus. Maybe we should look more closely at the marriage of Solomon and see the real Jesus. There is joy in heaven over repenting sinners; the family is glad when the prodigal son returns. Go forth and behold Jesus' grace toward sinners, as his crown, his brightest glory.

CHAPTER TWENTY-THREE

SONG OF SOLOMON 4:6 & 14

This chapter in Song of Solomon is about the same things that we have studied previously. I will quote the entire chapter from the <u>New American Standard Version</u> using **MYRRH** in two passages, since that is the reason why we are studying **MYRRH** ...

*"How beautiful you are, my darling, how beautiful you are! Your eyes are like doves behind your veil; your hair is like a flock of goats that have descended from Mount Gilead. 2 "Your teeth are like a flock of newly shorn ewes which have come up from their washing, all of which bear twins, and not one among them has lost her young. 3 "Your lips are like a scarlet thread, and your mouth is lovely. Your temples are like a slice of a pomegranate behind your veil. 4 "Your neck is like the tower of David built with rows of stone on which are hung a thousand shields all the round shields of the mighty men. 5 Your two breasts are like two fawns twins of a gazelle which feed among the lilies. 6 Until the cool of the day when the shadows flee away, I will go my way to the mountain of **MYRRH** and to the hill of **FRANKINCENSE**. 7 "You are altogether beautiful, my darling and there is no blemish in you. 8 "Come with me from Lebanon, my bride, may you come with me from Lebanon. Journey down from the summit of Amana, from the summit of Senir and Hermon, from the dens of lions, from the mountains of leopards. 9 "You have made my heart beat faster, my sister, my bride; you have made my heart beat faster with a single glance of your eyes, with a single strand of your*

*necklace. 10 How beautiful is your love, my sister, my bride! How much better is your love than wine, and the fragrance of your oils than all kinds of spices! 11 "Your lips, my bride, drip honey; honey and milk are under your tongue, and the fragrance of your garments is like the fragrance of Lebanon. 12 "A garden locked is my sister, my bride, a rock garden locked, a spring sealed up. 13 "Your shoots are an orchard of pomegranates with choice fruits, henna with nard plants, 14 Nard and saffron, calamus and cinnamon, with all the trees of **FRANKINCENSE, MYRRH** and aloes, along with all the finest spices. 15 "You are a garden spring, a well of fresh water and streams flowing from Lebanon." 16 "Awake, O north wind and come, wind of the south; make my garden breathe out fragrance, let its spices be wafted abroad. May my beloved come into his garden and eat its choice fruits!"*

Other than the word **FRANKINCENSE**, used twice and the word **MYRRH** mentioned three times, we have basically covered the verses before, so I will move along to the next verse.

CHAPTER TWENTY-FOUR

SONG OF SOLOMON 5:1 & 5

MYRRH is mentioned once in verse 1 and twice in verse 5. Here is the quotation from the <u>New American Standard Version</u> of the paragraph ...

*"I have come into my garden, my sister, my bride; I have gathered my **MYRRH** along with my balsam. I have eaten my honeycomb and my honey; I have drunk my wine and my milk. Eat, friends; drink and imbibe deeply, O lovers." 2 "I was asleep but my heart was awake. A voice! My beloved was knocking: 'Open to me, my sister, my darling, my dove, my perfect one! For my head is drenched with dew, my locks with the damp of the night.' 3 "I have taken off my dress, how can I put it on again? I have washed my feet, how can I dirty them again? 4 "My beloved extended his hand through the opening, and my feelings were aroused for him. 5 "I arose to open to my beloved; and my hands dripped with **MYRRH**, and my fingers with liquid **MYRRH**, on the handles of the bolt. 6 "I opened to my beloved, but my beloved had turned away and had gone! My heart went out to him as he spoke. I searched for him but I did not find him; I called him but he did not answer me. 7 "The watchmen who make the rounds in the city found me, they struck me and wounded me; the guardsmen of the walls took away my shawl from me. 8 "I adjure you, O daughters of Jerusalem, if you find my beloved, as to what you will tell him: For I am lovesick." 9 "What kind of beloved is your beloved, O most beautiful among women? What kind of beloved is your beloved, that thus you adjure us?"*

This series of verses deals with **<u>the torment of separation</u>** between the two lovers. However, it is still dealing with the handsomeness of the male and the loveliness of the wife so I will go on to the next scripture.

CHAPTER TWENTY-FIVE

SONG OF SOLOMON 5:13

The passage of scripture that is last about **MYRRH** is listed above on the heading. Here it is from the New American Standard Version ...

"My beloved is dazzling and ruddy, outstanding among ten thousand. 11 "His head is like gold, pure gold; his locks are like clusters of dates and black as a raven. 12 His eyes are like doves beside streams of water, bathed in milk, and reposed in their setting. 13 "His cheeks are like a bed of balsam, banks of sweet-scented herbs; his lips are lilies dripping with liquid MYRRH. 14 "His hands are rods of gold. Set with beryl his abdomen is carved ivory inlaid with sapphires. 15 "His legs are pillars of alabaster set on pedestals of pure gold; his appearance is like Lebanon choice as the cedars. 16 "His mouth is full of sweetness. And he is wholly desirable. This is my beloved and this is my friend, O daughters of Jerusalem."

This verse has **MYRRH** in verse 13 but this is the last one in the Bible. We have covered them all in both **MYRRH** and **FRANKINCENSE** along with other thoughts. This passage is mainly about the admiration by the bride. So, we will wind things up in the next two chapters.

CHAPTER TWENTY SIX

GOLD

The ~~three~~ wise men gave presents to Jesus in Nazareth about two years after he was born. If you have not seen that, you need to go back and read this book again.

In the tabernacle (*tent of meeting*), what was not covered with **GOLD**? The stories about **GOLD** goes all of the way through the Bible from Genesis through Revelation. We begin looking at it in the garden in Eden. The name of the first of five **rivers** that connected the garden was …

*"The name of the first is Pishon; it flows around the whole land of Havilah, where there is **GOLD**. 12 The **GOLD** of that land is good; the bdellium and the onyx stone are there"* [Genesis 2:11-12 NASU].

And then, we find many verses throughout the Bible and we wind up in Revelation. The last verse is about the New Jerusalem …

*"The one who spoke with me had a **GOLD** measuring rod to measure the city, and its gates and its wall. 16 The city is laid out as a square, and its length is as great as the width; and he measured the city with the rod, fifteen hundred miles; its length and width and height are equal. 17 And he measured its wall, seventy-two yards, according to human measurements, which are also angelic measurements. 18 The material of the wall was jasper; and the city was pure **GOLD**, like*

*clear glass. 19 The foundation stones of the city wall were adorned with every kind of precious stone. The first foundation stone was jasper; the second, sapphire; the third, chalcedony; the fourth, emerald; 20 the fifth, sardonyx; the sixth, sardius; the seventh, chrysolite; the eighth, beryl; the ninth, topaz; the tenth, chrysoprase; the eleventh, jacinth; the twelfth, amethyst. 21 And the twelve gates were twelve pearls; each one of the gates was a single pearl. **And the street of the city was pure GOLD, like transparent glass**"* (Revelation 21:18 NASU].

With *"zahabh,"* **GOLD** frequently occurs with other words which, translated, mean *"pure," "refined," "finest," "beaten"* and *"Ophir."* You will have to study those words because I do not have the time and place for them in this book. The same is true of many of the following. Other terms occurring are; *"fine gold,""charuts," "kethem,"* literally, *"carved out," "ceghor"* and *"betser."*

In the Bible, the sources definitely mentioned in the *"old testament"* are: Havilah, Ophir, Sheba and Arabia. We are not justified in locating any of those places too definitely. They probably all refer to some region of Arabia.

The late origin of the geological formation of Palestine and Syria precludes the possibility of **GOLD** being found in any quantities, so that the large quantities of **GOLD** used by the children of Israel in constructing their holy places was not the product of mines in the country, but was from **the spoil and taxes** taken from the inhabitants of the land, or brought with them from Egypt. This **GOLD** was probably mined in Egypt, India or possibly Arabia, and brought by the great caravan routes through Arabia to Syria, or by sea in the ships of Tyre. There is no doubt about the Egyptian sources. The old workings in the **GOLD**-bearing veins of the Egyptian desert and the ruins of the buildings connected with the mining and refining of the precious metal **still remain**. This region is being reopened with the prospect of its becoming a source of part of the world's supply. It might be inferred from the extensive spoils in **GOLD** taken from the Midianites (100,000 pounds, <u>Hastings, Dictionary of the Bible</u>) that their country of Northwestern Arabia produced **GOLD**. It is more likely that the Midianites had, in turn, **captured** most of it from other weaker nations. The tradition that Northwestern Arabia is rich in **GOLD** still persists. Every year, Moslem pilgrims, returning from Mecca by the Damascus route, bring with them specimens of **what is supposed** to be **GOLD** ore. They secure it from the Arabs at the stopping-places along the route. Samples analyzed have been **iron pyrites only**. No **GOLD**-bearing rock has yet appeared. Whether these specimens come from the mines mentioned by Burton is a question.

GOLD formed a part of every household treasure. It was probably treasured in the form of nuggets in regularly or irregularly shaped slabs or bars and in the form of dust. A specimen of yellow dust, which the owner claimed to have taken from an ancient jar, unearthed in the vicinity of the Hauran, was once brought to a laboratory. On examination, it was found to contain **iron pyrites** and metallic **GOLD** in a finely divided state. It was probably part of an ancient household treasure. A common practice was to make **GOLD** into jewelry with the dual purpose of ornamentation and of treasuring it. **This custom still prevails, especially among the Moslems, who do not let out their money at interest**. A poor woman will save her small coins until she has enough to buy a **GOLD** bracelet. This she will wear or put away against the day of need. It was weight and not beauty which was noted in the jewels. **GOLD coinage was unknown in the early "*old testament*" times.**

The use of **GOLD** as the most convenient way of treasuring wealth is mentioned above. Jewelry took many forms - armlets, bracelets, chains, crescents, crowns, earrings and rings. Making and decorating objects in connection with places of worship was also in **GOLD**. In the description of the building of the ark and the tabernacle in Exodus 25, we read of the lavish use of **GOLD** in **overlaying wood and metals**, and in shaping candlesticks, dishes, spoons, flagons, bowls, snuffers, curtain clasps, hooks, etc.. One estimate of the value of gold used is 90,000 pounds (see Hastings, Dictionary of the Bible). Other passages are records of still more extensive use of **GOLD** in building the temple. **GOLD** was used for lavish display. Even idols were built of **GOLD**. Among the fabulous luxuries of Solomon's court were his **GOLD** drinking-vessels, a throne of ivory overlaid with **GOLD**, and golden chariot trimmings. Sacred treasure saved from offerings or portions dedicated **from booty** were principally **GOLD**. This treasure was **the spoil** most sought after by the enemy. It was **paid to them as tribute** or taken as **plunder**.

As to its **FIGURATIVE** use in the Bible, **GOLD** is used to **symbolize** earthly riches that are finer than **GOLD**, which, physically speaking, is considered non-perishable, typifies incorruptibility. Refining of **GOLD** is a figure for **great purity** or a **test of stedfastness**. **GOLD** was the most valuable of metals. It stood for anything of great value, hence was most worthy for use in worshipping Yahweh, and the adornment of angels or saints. The head was called golden as being the most precious part of the body (compare *"the golden bowl,"* of Ecclesiastes 12:6). *"The golden city"* meant Babylon as did also *"the golden cup,"* sensuality. A crown of **GOLD** was synonymous with royal honor. Wearing of **GOLD** typified lavish adornment and worldly luxury. Comparing men to **GOLD** suggested their nobility.

CHAPTER TWENTY SEVEN

<u>GOLDEN</u>

The ~~three~~ wise men of the Bible may have been even wiser than we thought! Researchers now believe that not only were the Magi very special people, but they were very likely thought of as healers in their own time. The gifts that they brought to the infant Jesus were likely some of the most powerful herbal healing remedies available... and according to research, continue to be some of the most powerful on the planet today.

We've taken centuries-old knowledge of the healing properties of frankincense, myrrh and "gold" **<u>turmeric</u>** and combined them into one of the most potent new anti-inflammatory supplement systems known to man.

Using the capsules and the essential oils separately is highly effective, but using both together provides the ultimate *"1-2 punch"* of health benefits! That's because applying the essential oils topically enables maximum absorption through the skin, while taking the capsules enables maximum absorption through your body's internal pathways. You can stop the root cause of all disease. One of the most powerful 1-2-3 punches to combat chronic inflammation in the world are **<u>Gold</u>**(en), Frankincense and Myrrh!

Your choice of topical, internal or **BOTH** – the ultra-pure essential oils provide the health benefits through your skin absorption, the capsule through your body's internal pathways … or for the ultimate in health benefits you can choose to use both! They can help maintain healthy gut function. Man has taken centuries-old knowledge of the healing properties of frankincense, myrrh and ***GOLD*** **turmeric** and combined them into one of the most potent new anti-inflammatory supplement systems known to man. Doctors across the globe are discovering gold, frankincense, and myrrh hold a little-known **secondary meaning** that could change the way we think about sickness forever. It could prevent nearly all chronic diseases (by stopping the source!): Get drug-free pain relief: Optimize one key process for better overall health!

You likely know the story of how the Magi brought the baby Jesus gifts of **gold**, frankincense, and myrrh after his birth. But what you **might not know** is how the hidden meaning behind these three gifts could have a proven and massive impact on your health, as well as the health of every other human on the face of the planet.

There are/were lifesaving health secrets hidden in the Magi's gifts. Biblical experts have countless interpretations of the Magi's three gifts, and there is indeed significance behind what was bestowed upon Jesus at his birth. However, groundbreaking research into the medicinal powers of the Magi's gifts, suggest that there might be far more to the symbolic meaning behind the age-old account of Jesus' birth than we ever imagined.

They were the real reason why these gifts were fit for the king. In Biblical times, **gold**, frankincense and myrrh were considered as treasured gifts fit for the utmost of royalty. That's why the Magi chose them for Jesus. But, the story runs far deeper than that, though. These three items weren't simply valued for their scarcity or expense (although they are still costly and difficult to find today). Rather, they were highly sought after for their unrivaled ability to control one key process in the body, which we know today to be the root cause behind nearly every ailment. How did the Magi know this?

Often mistranslated as *"King"* or *"Wise Man,"* the Greek word *"Magi"* means something very different from what you probably learned in your church. Actually, *"Magi"* is where we get the English words *"magic"* and *"magician,"* and the root meanings are much the same. Further, the Magi are said to have been traveling to see Jesus from *"the East,"* a region of the world known at the time for its great knowledge of natural remedies. So what did these revered men from the East know about **gold**, frankincense and myrrh that the rest of us might not? They were bearers of ancient Eastern wisdom.

Now we know that at least two of the three gifts of the Magi - frankincense and myrrh - possessed incredible medicinal powers. What's more, many argue that the third gift of **gold** could actually have been the *"golden spice"* of **turmeric**, which has its own set of amazing benefits. Together, these three gifts -- frankincense, myrrh, and turmeric -- represent a healing synergy that can be found nowhere else in nature. It appears that we have rediscovered the Magi's potent natural healers. The Magi understood this fact well, and that's part of the reason why they brought these three presents of inflammation to Jesus at his birth. And they knew how controlling inflammation could save your life.

Have you been struggling with chronic health problems, yet can't seem to figure out their source? Maybe you've endured a shocking diagnosis of something like cancer, heart disease or arthritis. Or perhaps you just look back on your younger days and realize you've felt *"off"* for years now, all the while never fully understanding where things went wrong.

Well, what does it take to properly control inflammation? Unfortunately, it's difficult to reap the full benefits of these three incredible plant substances -- turmeric, frankincense, and myrrh -- by consuming them in their natural state. They must be refined into an **extract** to offer the potent **medicinal** power you've just learned about. That's why the Magi brought them in the form of **gum and resin**, not just raw plant material. Considering the specific processing needed to maximize their medicinal value, as well as their scarcity, you're probably starting to think there's no way to take all three of these herbs together, extracted correctly, and without spending an arm and a leg.

Well, man has found a way of disarming cancer's #1 weapon before it even has a chance to strike. Cancer claims the lives of millions every year, and modern medicine still struggles to treat it effectively. Conventional physicians can do nothing else but resort to the same old toxic and invasive treatments - chemo, radiation and surgery. But what if man has found a way to fend off cancer before it has the chance to steal more innocent lives? If we could pinpoint the underlying culprit, it would give us priceless insight toward fighting cancer like we've never been able to before. Amazingly, many doctors seem to be doing just that, and their conclusions are raising a big red flag around the role of chronic inflammation in cancer.

There appears to be a new heart disease risk that most people still don't know. People of a certain age understand just how real the dangers of heart disease are.

We've seen it take friends, neighbors and family members. No surprise, considering it's the #1 cause of death in the United States, even over cancer. You may already be watching your blood pressure and cholesterol levels. If they're within an acceptable range, you're probably not that worried. But that may change when you learn how **recent** studies are revealing a **third** major risk factor nearly nobody's talking about or getting tested for at the doctor. According to Harvard, inflammation is the smoking gun behind a whole host of cardiovascular conditions. *"Chronic low-grade inflammation is intimately involved in all stages of atherosclerosis, the process that leads to cholesterol-clogged arteries. This means that inflammation sets the stage for heart attacks, most strokes, peripheral artery disease, and even vascular dementia, a common cause of memory loss."*

That means we're now being forced to entirely re-examine how we think about heart disease and the things that cause it. While things like cholesterol and blood pressure may be important, new evidence is suggesting they could just be manifestations of a deeper problem in the body - chronic inflammation.

While researchers are beginning to understand the core role inflammation plays in modern disease, they're looking in all the wrong places for a solution to it. Now that the connection between inflammation and disease is established, they'll spend millions of dollars trying to create anti-inflammatory **drugs** that will be expensive, hard-to-get, and riddled with side-effects. Meanwhile, those who **understand the gifts of the Magi** will be thrilled to know that the most potent inflammation controlling agents exist already! It can be obtained now in capsules or in essential oils at www.EpigeneticLabs.com, the only one of which I know.

CONCLUSION

I do not need to remind you of one passage in my book. Here it is as I remind you that the wise men gave gifts to Jesus …

> "*When they saw the star, they rejoiced exceedingly with great joy. 11 After coming into the house they saw the child with Mary his mother; and they fell to the ground and worshiped him. Then, opening their treasures, they presented to him gifts of **gold, frankincense, and myrrh**"* [Matthew 2:10-12].

Mainly, I wanted you to know of the precious oil and perfume that was given. **MYRRH** was very expensive and it was to be for **medicine** in Jesus' age.

Secondly, I wanted you to know of the Bible's use of **FRANKINCENSE**, that it was used for **medicine** too. It was more expensive than **MYRRH**.

GOLD (golden) was used for medicine. All three gifts were very expensive and could be used by Jesus in his physical body.

All three are expensive in today's world – 2017 A.D.. But learn about it, it will help your body to overcome all of your illness.

Thank you for reading this book!

RON McRAY

BOOKS BY RON MCRAY

- **The Last Days**
- **Through The Water, Through The Fire**
- **Behold, I Am Making All Things New**
- **Behold, I Am Coming Quickly**
- **Pearls Of Great Price**
- **What In The "World" Happened Between 30 A.D. And 70 A.D?**
- **The Lazarus Affair: A novel**
- **Did Jesus Have Long Hair?: The Biblical Verdict**
- **The Heavens Declare The Glory Of God: A Lost Understanding Of The Ancient Zodiac**
- **Was Jesus 3 Days And 3 Nights In The Heart Of The Earth?**
- **Satan, The Devil And The Adversary**
- **666 And The Anti-Christ Of Revelation**
- **God Came Riding On A Cloud**
- **The Good Life: A Biblical Understanding Of Being Spirit Filled**
- **Is It Wine Or Is It Grape Juice?**
- **The LORD Is Not Slack: Did God Keep His Promises… On Time?**
- **And We Think GOD Doesn't Talk To Us?**
- **The Judean Social Life**

- **Israel In Perspective**
- **Seeking Truth: The Scope And Sequence Of The Bible**
- **Are You In The Eternal Kingdom Of YAHWEH?**
- **Don't Worry About It Right Now**
- **Prophecy In 2017**
- **Real Medicine In Jesus' Day**

15 Book Series:

<u>Things That Your Preacher Forgot To Tell You!</u>

1. Righteousness Apart From Salvation: In The 1st Century
2. Is The Church The "ekklesia" Of The Bible?
3. Who Saw Jesus And When Did They See Him From His Crucifixion To His Ascension – And Why Is This So Important?
4. Are There Three Heavens – Or More?
5. Is It Appointed Unto Man Once To Die?
6. The Relationship Of The Church, The Kingdom And House To Eschatology
7. A Study Of Old Testament Prophets And Their Fulfillment
8. How To Interpret The Book Of Revelation Consistently
9. The Sign Of The End Revealed (Matthew 23,24,25)

10. Things That Were "About To Happen" In The Days Of Jesus And His Disciples
11. Someone Changed My Bible!
12. Ephesians: Not The Book That You Thought That It Was
13. The Lord's Supper
14. First-Born And Second-Born: A Study Of Types and Anti-types
15. The Writings Of Jesus Revealed!

DVD'S BY DR. RON MCRAY

- **Introduction To Eschatology**
- **Why Am I Here – What Is My Purpose?**

Use this link to access the website for all information concerning books

www.EschatologyReview.com

Toll-free ordering 1-888-393-5933

Be sure to get your free audio book here:

www.EschatologyReview.com/b1